MW01414803

DOT Medical Exams: The Complete Guide

J. J. Keller
& Associates, Inc.®
Since 1953

Copyright 2013

J. J. Keller & Associates, Inc.
3003 Breezewood Lane, P.O. Box 368
Neenah, Wisconsin 54957-0368
Phone: (800) 327-6868
Fax: (800) 727-7516
JJKeller.com

Library of Congress Catalog Card Number: 2013930746

ISBN: 978-61099-413-2

Canadian Goods and Services Tax (GST) Number: R123-317687

First Edition, Ninth Printing, April 2022

TABLE OF CONTENTS

Introduction

A safe driver is a healthy driver. That's one reason the Federal Motor Carrier Safety Administration (FMCSA) – as the federal agency in charge of truck and bus safety – sets standards for the physical and mental condition of the nation's commercial motor vehicle drivers.

Through regular physical examinations, commercial drivers are required to demonstrate that they're fit for duty and won't pose a danger to themselves or the traveling public.

From drug use and poor vision to hypertension and diabetes, the list of ailments and conditions that can disqualify a driver is long, but not as long as the list of those harmed or killed by drivers who were unfit to be behind the wheel.

Consider, for example, the case of a Mother's Day accident in New Orleans involving a fully loaded motorcoach. The driver lost consciousness on an interstate highway and crashed the bus into an embankment, killing 22 passengers and seriously injuring himself and another 15 passengers. Investigators found that the driver had multiple, serious medical conditions which his employer and healthcare providers all knew about, including end-stage kidney failure and congestive heart failure. The driver had seen *dozens* of healthcare providers over the previous two years. Unfortunately, he was given a medical certificate nine months prior to the accident, in spite of the obviously disqualifying medical problems.

This accident and others like it are preventable, and that's where this *Guide* comes in. It was designed to:

• Help transportation safety professionals understand the complex federal medical standards and driver examination process, from head to toe;

1

- Serve as a handy reference guide for the many medical issues that could derail a driver's career;

- Help resolve the many conflicts, complications, and other problems that can arise before, during, and after a DOT medical exam;

- Help comply with challenging recordkeeping requirements; and

- Help drivers stay in shape and pass their next medical exam, or obtain waivers or exemptions when they cannot.

> An estimated 3 to 4 million DOT driver physical exams are performed annually.

Does This Guide Apply to You?

This guide is based on the federal medical standards found in 49 CFR Part 391, Subpart E, of the Federal Motor Carrier Safety Regulations. These standards apply to drivers of "commercial motor vehicles," being any vehicle used on a public road in interstate commerce when the vehicle or combination of vehicles:

- Weighs or is rated at 10,001 pounds (4,536 kg) or more;

- Is used to haul hazardous materials in a quantity that requires a placard;

- Is designed or used to transport 16 or more passengers (including the driver); or

- Is designed or used to transport 9 or more passengers (including the driver) for direct compensation.

Refer to Chapter 2 for more details.

Note: Because this guide is based primarily on federal rules, it does not contain complete details on state laws or regulations for driver qualification, although they are often the same.

The section symbol (§) is used to designate a section of the Federal Motor Carrier Safety Regulations as found in Title 49 of the Code of Federal Regulations. Some of those regulations may be found in Chapter 9.

KEEP IN MIND: This guide is meant for educational reference only and is not intended to provide legal or medical advice. Do not attempt to diagnose or treat any medical condition without seeking help from a medical professional. Only a medical examiner is qualified to determine if a driver is medically qualified to operate a commercial motor vehicle.

Due to the constantly changing nature of the FMCSA medical qualification process, regulations, and guidelines, a website has been created to keep you informed of any forthcoming changes affecting this *Guide*. For the latest information, go to:
jjkeller.com/DMEH

I. DOT Exams at a Glance

Who Needs a DOT Medical Exam?

- Any interstate driver who operates a "commercial motor vehicle" (CMV) as defined in §390.5.

- Any intrastate-only driver operating a vehicle that requires placarding for hazardous materials.

- Any intrastate-only driver who is required to comply with the medical examination requirements under his/her state's laws or regulations.

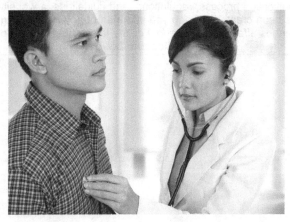

When Is a DOT Exam Required?

- Before first operating a CMV;

- At least every two years, or more often as directed by the medical examiner; and

- Whenever the driver's ability to perform his or her normal duties has been impaired by a physical or mental injury or disease.

Who Can Perform an Exam?

Anyone currently listed on the National Registry of Certified Medical Examiners — online at nationalregistry.fmcsa.dot.gov — may perform an exam for an interstate driver. This may include medical doctors, osteopaths, physician assistants, advanced practice nurses, and chiropractors. State requirements may vary for intrastate-only drivers.

What Are the Basic Medical Standards?

AREA	STANDARD	
Diabetes	No diabetes controlled with insulin unless the driver qualifies under §391.46.	
Blood pressure	**BP Reading**	**Status**
	<140/90	Qualified
	140-159/90-99	Qualified for 1 year
	160-179/100-109	Qualified for 3 months
	≥180/110	Disqualified
Vision*	• Distant vision of at least 20/40 in each eye without corrective lenses OR separately corrected to 20/40 or better with corrective lenses; • Distant binocular vision of at least 20/40 in both eyes with or without corrective lenses; • Field of vision of at least 70 degrees in the horizontal meridian in each eye; and • Ability to recognize red, yellow, and green traffic signals. • Drivers not meeting this standard may qualify for up to 1 year, based on vision in the better eye, under the alternate vision standard in §391.44.	
Hearing*	• First perceives a forced whispered voice in the better ear at not less than 5 feet, with or without the use of a hearing aid; OR • If tested with an audiometric device, does not have an average hearing loss in the better ear greater than 40 decibels, with or without a hearing aid.	

AT A GLANCE

I. DOT Exams at a Glance

AREA	STANDARD
Respiratory system	No respiratory problem that could lead to unsafe driving.
Vascular (blood) system	No cardiovascular disease known to be associated with fainting, breathing difficulties, collapse, or heart failure.
Limbs	No loss of a foot, leg, hand, or arm, and no impairmont of a hand, finger, arm, foot, or leg which interferes with normal tasks, unless granted a Skill Performance Evaluation (SPE) certificate.
Joints/bones/ muscles	No rheumatic, arthritic, orthopedic, muscular, neuromuscular, or vascular disease which interferes with safe driving ability.
Epilepsy*	No epilepsy or any other condition likely to cause loss of consciousness or loss of vehicle control.
Psychiatric	No mental, nervous, organic, or functional disease or psychiatric disorder likely to lead to unsafe driving.
Drugs	Does not use any Schedule I drug, amphetamine, narcotic, or any other habit-forming drug. Limited exceptions exist for certain prescriptions (see below).
Alcohol	Is not diagnosed as an alcoholic.

*The standards for vision, hearing, and epilepsy are absolute "non-discretionary" standards, meaning the examiner does not have discretion to qualify someone who does not meet the objective standards for those conditions. A driver who is not able to comply with those standards must obtain a waiver in order to drive in interstate commerce. Drivers using insulin may only be certified under the terms of §391.46. The remaining nine standards are "discretionary" standards and the medical examiner can make a clinical judgment concerning qualification.

Which Drugs Are Disqualifying?

Drivers can never take drugs identified in Schedule I, even with a prescription. Other drugs that are disqualifying include:

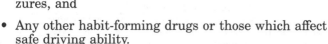

- Amphetamines,

- Narcotics (including methadone),

- Insulin to control diabetes (except as allowed in §391.46),

- Any anti-seizure medication used for the prevention of seizures, and

- Any other habit-forming drugs or those which affect safe driving ability.

Exceptions: Drivers can take non-Schedule I drugs if the prescribing doctor documents that the driver is safe to be a commercial driver while taking the medication. In that case, the medical examiner may – but does not have to – certify the driver. The medical examiner may make his/her own determination that the medication is safe, or may request a letter from the prescribing doctor. Insulin use is allowed if the driver qualifies under the terms of §391.46.

A driver cannot take a controlled substance or prescription medication without a prescription from a licensed practitioner. Also note that under §383.51, CDL-licensed drivers who are convicted of being under the influence of any controlled substance listed in Schedules I-V may lose their driving privileges.

Refer to the subject index at the back of this Guide for information on specific medications. See also Chapter 9 for the complete Schedules of Controlled Substances.

AT A GLANCE

Which Records Need to Be Kept?

There are several types of documents that may be generated in connection with a driver's medical qualification, each with their own retention requirements. See Chapter 5 for additional details. Note that state requirements may vary for intrastate drivers.

Document	Description	Retention
Medical Examination Report (a.k.a., "long form," MCSA-5875)	This 5-page form (8-9 pages with instructions) is completed by the driver and medical examiner during the exam. It includes a health history and results of the exam, as well as instructions for completing the form. It may be paper or electronic.	Retained in the medical examiner's office for at least 3 years. Under medical privacy laws (HIPAA), the form may not be released to employers without consent of the driver.
Medical Examiner's Certificate (a.k.a., wallet card, med card, fed-med card, MCSA-5876)	This one-page certificate must be completed by the medical examiner if the driver is medically qualified to drive.* The certificate expires at midnight on the expiration day shown on the certificate; there is no grace period. Interstate CDL/CLP drivers need to provide the original or a copy to their state licensing agency (check with licensing agency for details).	Original provided to driver, to be kept until it expires. Motor carrier must retain copy for 3 years, unless required to use MVR instead (see §391.51(a)(7)). Medical examiner retains a copy for at least 3 years, and must provide copy to driver's current or prospective motor-carrier employer(s) upon request. State licensing agency retains for at least 3 years, if applicable.
CMV Driver Medical Examination Results Form (MCSA-5850)	This is an electronic form that medical examiners use to report exam results to the FMCSA. It is submitted via the examiner's personal National Registry web account.	—

Document	Description	Retention
391.41 CMV Driver Medication Form (MCSA-5895)	This is an optional form for medical examiners to request additional information from a driver's treating physician concerning any medications the driver might be taking and the medical conditions being treated with those medications.	Retained in the medical examiner's office for at least 3 years.
Insulin-Treated Diabetes Mellitus Assessment Form (MCSA-5870)	This 4-page form is completed by the treating clinician for a driver who is using insulin to control diabetes mellitus. Within 45 days of the form's completion, the driver must bring it to his/her next scheduled DOT medical exam.	Retained in the medical examiner's office for at least 3 years.
Vision Evaluation Report (MCSA-5871)	The driver must present to the Medical Examiner, a completed Vision Evaluation Report, Form MCSA–5871, that is signed and dated by an ophthalmologist or optometrist not more than 45 days prior to the medical exam.	Retained in the medical examiner's office for at least 3 years.
Motor Vehicle Record (a.k.a., MVR, driving record)	The driving records of **interstate CDL/CLP drivers** must contain the driver's current medical certification status. The motor carrier must obtain the MVR and verify the driver's status before he/she drives (or a copy of the med card can be used instead, for up to 15 days from the card's issuance date). A new MVR must be obtained each time the driver obtains a new med card.	Retained by motor carrier for 3 years. MVR obtained at time of hire must be kept until 3 years after employment ends.

AT A GLANCE

9

Document	Description	Retention
Skill Performance Evaluation Certificate (a.k.a., SPE certificate)	This certificate is issued to drivers who have impaired or missing limbs and who have been granted a waiver under §391.49.	Original retained by driver until it expires. Copy retained by employing motor carrier for 3 years from issuance date.
Medical waiver, variance, or exemption	Documentation that a driver has received a waiver, variance, or exemption from one or more medical qualification rules. These may be issued by the FMCSA or by a state enforcement agency.	Retained by driver until it expires. Copy retained by employer for 3 years from issuance date. State retention requirements may vary.
Verification of National Registry listing	The motor carrier must verify and document (via a "note") that the driver's medical examiner was listed on the National Registry of Certified Medical Examiners at the time of the exam.*	Retained in driver qualification file for 3 years.

*Beginning June 23, 2025, medical exam certificates will not have to be issued to CDL/CLP drivers. The MVR will be the only acceptable proof that a CDL/CLP driver is medically certified. In addition, there will be no need to verify that the CDL/CLP driver's medical examiner is listed on the National Registry.

II. Overview

Who Has to Comply?

The federal DOT medical standards – found in Part 391 of the Federal Motor Carrier Safety Regulations – apply to anyone who drives a commercial motor vehicle, or CMV, as defined in federal regulations. A vehicle is considered a CMV if it meets these criteria:

It is a motor vehicle. This means it's a truck, bus, tractor, trailer, semitrailer, or any other vehicle or machine that is propelled or drawn by mechanical power to transport passengers or property. This does not include vehicles operated exclusively on rails, nor certain types of off-road construction equipment.

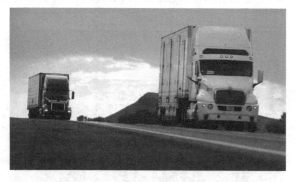

It is of a certain size OR hauls hazmat. The "CMV" label is not limited to class 8 trucks or large buses. A vehicle is large enough to be a CMV if it either:

- Weighs or is rated* at 10,001 pounds or more (including all vehicles in the combination, if there is more than one); OR

- Is used *or designed* to transport 9 or more passengers (including the driver) and there is direct compensation involved ("direct compensation" is payment

11

made to the motor carrier by the passengers or a person acting on behalf of the passengers for the transportation services provided, and not included in a total package charge or other assessment for highway transportation services); OR

- Is used *or designed* to transport 16 or more passengers (including the driver) and is not used to transport passengers for compensation.

No matter what size the vehicle is, if it is used to transport hazardous materials in a quantity that requires placards, then it is automatically a CMV.

*NOTE: The vehicle rating is based on the heavier of the gross vehicle weight rating (GVWR) or the gross combination weight rating (GCWR). If not marked on the vehicle, the GCWR can be determined by adding together the actual weight or GVWRs of the power unit and trailer.

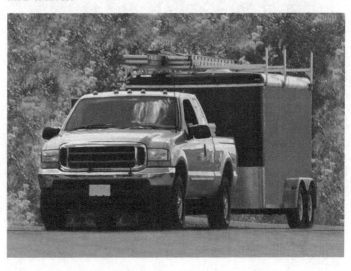

It is used on a "highway." The term "highway" includes much more than the interstates. A highway is any road, street, or way that is open to public travel, even if it's on private property. "Open to public travel" means that the area is accessible to standard passenger cars and is open to the general public for use, which could include a private parking lot or private road, for example. If there are restrictive gates, prohibitive signs, or other restrictions on travel, then it may not be considered a highway (toll roads are highways even if they have toll gates).

It is used in commerce. "Commerce" means the buying and selling of goods and services. It also deals with moving those goods from place to place or going somewhere to perform the service. Any work done in support of a business is considered to be commerce. Even a church that provides bus tours to the general public for compensation is considered to be operating in commerce.

Specifically, it is used in* interstate *commerce. *Interstate* commerce means the goods have traveled into or through another state or country or someone has gone into another state or country to perform the service. Even if your vehicle does not leave your state, but the goods or services have or will, then the transportation within your state is usually considered to be interstate commerce. For example:

- If a shipper is sending a "widget" to another state or into your state and you transport it part of the way but you never leave your state, your part of the move is still considered interstate commerce.

- If you drive an empty vehicle into another state to move cargo or passengers within that state, it's interstate commerce.

When operating in interstate commerce, you have to follow the *federal* driver qualification rules. On the other hand, if your vehicles, goods, and services stay within a single state, then you may be engaged in "intrastate" commerce and are subject to your state's rules. In most cases, the state rules mirror the federal rules – especially for drivers hauling a placarded amount of hazardous materials – but there are exceptions. In some cases, those exceptions depend on the types of cargo or number of passengers being carried or the size of the vehicle. Consult state laws and regulations for details.

A Pickup Truck Can Be a CMV!

Many people assume that smaller vehicles like pickup trucks are automatically exempt from the rules, especially when they are used by a private company, don't have air brakes, don't require a commercial driver's license (CDL), and stay close to home. But many pickups and small straight trucks, especially when used to pull a trailer, are regulated as CMVs because they are used for a business and they exceed the 10,000-pound threshold.

Complete this four-part test to see if your pickup is a CMV:

1. Look at the manufacturer's rating plate. Is the gross vehicle weight rating (GVWR) 10,001 pounds or more?

2. Look at the GVWR of the trailer(s) that are pulled with that truck, if any, and add that to the GVWR of the truck. Does it add up to 10,001 pounds or more?

3. When the vehicle (truck and trailer) is fully loaded with fuel and cargo and/or people, does it actually weigh 10,001 pounds or more when driven over a scale?

4. Do you ever transport enough hazardous materials that you need to put a placard on the vehicle?

If you answered "yes" to any of these questions, then the vehicle is a CMV and you probably have to comply with the federal DOT medical exam standards (and lots of other safety rules), especially if you cross state lines. If you stay within a single state, then you may be exempt in that state.

What if you unhook the trailer and can answer "no" to all four questions? Then the truck by itself is not a CMV under federal rules and the driver may be exempt from needing a medical exam.

What About the Type of "Cargo"?

Notice that the definition of commercial motor vehicle makes no mention of what the vehicle is carrying, except in the case of hazmat and passenger vehicles. Whether the vehicle is carrying cargo, commodities, tools, equipment, supplies, or even nothing at all, it can still be considered a CMV.

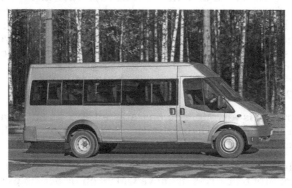

9- to 15-Passenger Vans

Drivers of limos, vans, or other passenger-carrying vehicles that were designed to carry 9 to 15 passengers may or may not be subject to the medical exam rules. If a vehicle weighs or is rated at less than 10,001 pounds and there is no "direct compensation," then the vehicle

OVERVIEW

may qualify for the exemption under §390.3(f)(6) and the driver would not have to comply with DOT medical standards.

There is "direct compensation" if the passengers (or a person acting on behalf of the passengers) pay the driver or company for the transportation service being provided, and the payment is not included in a total package charge or other assessment for highway transportation services.

If the vehicles weigh or are rated at 10,001 pounds or more, regardless of compensation, then the rules apply due to the weight alone. If the vehicles weigh less than 10,001 pounds and there is no compensation of any kind for the transportation (such as a company transporting its own employees), then the vehicles are exempt.

If a driver is subject to the Part 391 rules but the company is classified as a non-business private motor carrier of passengers (such as a church group, scout group, or other charitable organization transporting its own members in a 9- to 15-passenger van), then the driver is exempt from needing a medical exam or medical certificate.

Who Is a "Driver"?

A "driver" is anyone who operates a CMV at any time, even if it's not in their job title. The following are all drivers who may need a medical exam:

* Mechanics or other shop personnel who may occasionally test-drive or move CMVs on or across public roadways.

* Managers, supervisors, the company owner or president, or other personnel who may get behind the wheel of a CMV and take it onto a public roadway.

* Owner-operators, part-time drivers, driver trainees, full-time drivers, or anyone else who drives a CMV.

Drivers From Canada and Mexico

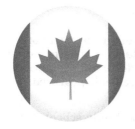

Drivers based in Canada and Mexico who carry a commercial driver's license (CDL) from their home country but drive commercial vehicles in the U.S. do not necessarily need to have a medical exam in the U.S.

The reciprocity agreement applies to the "Licencia Federal de Conductor" issued by the United Mexican States and CDLs issued by Canadian provinces or territories. Canadian and Mexican CMV drivers are not required to carry proof of medical certification as long as their license and medical status, including any waiver or exemption, can be electronically verified. Drivers with a Canadian Class 5, Ontario Class G, Ontario Class D (prior to age 80), New Brunswick Class 3 license (prior to age 65), or Alberta Class 3 license must provide additional documentation (letter, U.S. med card, or endorsement code).

Be aware that there may be cases where a medical waiver or variance will not be accepted in the United States. According to U.S. regulations, drivers "who have received a medical authorization that deviates from the mutually accepted compatible medical standards of the resident country are not qualified to drive a CMV in

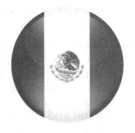

the other countries." For example, Canadian drivers who do not meet the medical fitness provisions of the Canadian National Safety Code for Motor Carriers, but are issued a waiver by one of the Canadian Provinces or Territories, are not qualified to drive a CMV in the United States. In addition, U.S. drivers who received a medical variance from the FMCSA are not qualified to drive a CMV in Canada.

OVERVIEW

17

Exemptions

FMCSR Exemptions

The following drivers are exempt from all or parts of the Federal Motor Carrier Safety Regulations, including the medical standards. There are additional exemptions from just the medical standards specifically, covered below.

- **School bus drivers** who transport only school children and/or school personnel from home to school and from school to home.

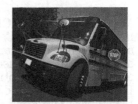

- Drivers working directly for the federal **government**, a state, or any political subdivision of a state. This does not apply to motor carriers simply doing business with the government.

- Drivers who use a CMV to "occasionally" transport **personal property**, as long as it is not done for compensation or for a commercial purpose.

- Drivers who occasionally use CMVs to transport cars, boats, horses, etc., to **races, tournaments, shows**, or similar events are exempt IF the underlying activities are not done for profit (that is, for tax purposes, the prize money is declared as ordinary income and the cost of the underlying activities is not deducted as a business expense) and there is no corporate sponsorship.

- Drivers who transport human **corpses or sick or injured persons**.

- Drivers operating **fire trucks and rescue vehicles** while involved in emergency operations.

- Drivers operating CMVs designed or used to transport between **9 and 15 passengers** (including the driver) when there is no direct compensation and the vehicles are not over 10,000 pounds or hauling a placarded amount of hazardous materials.

- Drivers of CMVs used primarily in the transportation of **propane winter heating fuel** or used to respond to a **pipeline emergency**, if the regulations would prevent the driver from responding to an "emergency condition requiring immediate response" as defined in §390.5 (this does not include requests to refill empty gas tanks).

- Drivers providing **emergency relief** during a declared emergency (§390.23).

- Drivers of **off-road motorized construction equipment**, not including mobile cranes. This is limited to equipment which (by its design and function) is obviously not intended for use on a public road. The exemption applies when operated at construction sites and when operated on a public road as long as the equipment is not used in furtherance of a transportation purpose.

Medical Qualification Exemptions

The following drivers may be eligible for an exemption from the medical qualification standards, even though other DOT safety regulations may still apply:

Applies To	Description	Rule
Drivers furnished by other motor carriers	If a driver is regularly employed and fully qualified by one motor carrier, he or she can perform work for another motor carrier without presenting his or her medical certificate as long as the regularly employing carrier gives the other motor carrier a signed, written statement certifying that the driver is qualified.	§391.65

OVERVIEW

Applies To	Description	Rule
Farm vehicles	Most of Part 391 does not apply to farm vehicle drivers unless driving articulated (combination) vehicles. See definitions in §390.5 (see Chapter 9).	§391.2(c)
Covered farm vehicles	The medical standards in 49 CFR 391, Subpart E, do not apply to drivers of "covered" farm vehicles. See definition in §390.5 (see Chapter 9).	§391.2(d)
Custom harvesting	Most of Part 391 does not apply to vehicles used to transport farm machinery, supplies, or both, to or from a farm for custom-harvesting operations on a farm; or to transport custom-harvested crops to storage or market.	§391.2(a)
Beekeepers	Most of Part 391 does not apply to drivers operating vehicles controlled and operated by a beekeeper engaged in the seasonal transportation of bees.	§391.2(b)
Private motor carrier of passengers (nonbusiness)	Drivers for nonbusiness, private motor carriers of passengers are exempt from the requirements to be medically examined and to carry a medical certificate.	§391.68
Intra-city zone drivers	The medical standards in §391.41(b), except those related to drug/alcohol abuse, do not apply to those who drove a CMV in a municipality or exempt intracity zone throughout the one-year period ending November 18, 1988, and whose medical condition has not substantially worsened since then.	§391.62
Drivers participating in vision waiver study program or using a federal vision exemption	The vision standards do not apply to drivers who were participating in a vision waiver study program as of March 31, 1996. NOTE: Medical cards issued under the vision waiver study program will be void on and after March 22, 2023. Individuals physically qualified under the grandfather provision in §391.64(b) or a federal vision exemption have until 11:59 P.M. March 21, 2023, to comply with the alternate vision standard in §391.44.	§391.64

Exemptions for Specific Medical Issues

Federal exemptions — The FMCSA offers several
types of special exemptions or waivers for specific conditions. These exemptions are valid for up to two years
and can be renewed. Exemptions can only be issued by
a regulatory agency; medical examiners cannot issue
exemptions. Additional details may be found below and
in Chapter 6.

- **Diabetes:** Drivers with insulin-treated diabetes mellitus (ITDM) must follow the procedures in §391.46
  to become medically certified. The ITDM exemption
  program that began in 2003 was withdrawn in February 2019. Drivers who still hold an exemption
  must use the new process outlined in §391.46 before
  their medical certificate expires.

- **Vision:** Drivers who do not meet the vision standard
  (§391.41(b)(10)) may qualify under the alternate vision standard in §391.44 on and after March 22,
  2022. Medical cards issued under the vision waiver
  study program or a federal vision exemption will be
  void on and after March 22, 2023. Individuals physically qualified under the grandfather provisions in §
  391.64(b) or a federal vision exemption have until
  11:59 P.M. March 21, 2023, to comply with the alternate vision standard in §391.44.

> Additional information about federal medical exemptions
> can be obtained by e-mail to medicalexemptions@dot.gov
> or fmcsamedical@dot.gov. Certain exemption applications
> are available on the FMCSA website.

- **Hearing:** On a case-by-case basis, the FMCSA is issuing exemptions from its hearing standard
  (§391.41(b)(11)). More information and forms for applying for this exemption are available on the
  FMCSA website. Hearing-impaired drivers who receive an exemption have to get annual medical
  exams and cannot operate buses with passengers on
  board.

OVERVIEW

21

- **Epilepsy/seizures:** Drivers with a history of epilepsy, seizure(s), or other conditions likely to cause a loss of ability to control a CMV can apply for an exemption from the epilepsy standard (§391.41(b)(8)). More information and forms for applying for this exemption are available on the FMCSA website.

- **Limb disorders:** Drivers with physical impairments affecting their ability to safely operate CMVs (as determined by their medical examiner) or with missing limbs (e.g., hand, finger, arm, foot, or leg), are required to obtain Skill Performance Evaluation (SPE) certificates. Applicants have to demonstrate safe driving ability. An application is available on the FMCSA website or by contacting an FMCSA Service Center. The state of Virginia is also authorized to issue SPE certificates for interstate drivers.

> The federal exemptions above apply to drivers who intend to operate CMVs in *interstate* commerce; the FMCSA has no authority to grant a waiver/exemption from a state's in-state requirements.

State exemptions — Individual states can grant exemptions to drivers involved in intrastate commerce, as long as those drivers do not cross state lines or otherwise get involved in interstate commerce. Vision and diabetes waivers are not uncommon, and states often have "grandfathering" provisions as well. Contact the state's CMV enforcement agency for details.

When Is a DOT Medical Exam Required?

Before a driver can drive a commercial motor vehicle, he or she must first pass a DOT medical exam and be issued a Medical Examiner's Certificate, commonly known as a "med card" or "wallet card."

The employing motor carrier must have proof that the driver is medically qualified before allowing him or her to operate a CMV in commerce. This proof can result from a new medical exam at the time of hire or from a driver's previous exam if that exam is still valid.

In addition, a new medical card must be obtained:

• At least every two years, or more often as directed by the medical examiner. Medical cards can be valid for no more than two years but expire sooner due to medical conditions, at the discretion of the examiner.

• Whenever the driver's ability to perform his or her normal duties has been impaired by a physical or mental injury or disease. It is a shared responsibility between the motor carrier and driver to determine when these conditions exist.

> A driver who is unable to pass a DOT medical exam must not drive commercial vehicles until he or she is able to pass the exam or obtain a waiver or exemption!

Q: My driver's new medical card is only valid for 1 year (or 6 months, or 3 months, etc.). How is that possible?
A: Two years is the *maximum* certification period, but there is no minimum. The examiner has discretion to certify drivers for a shorter period of time if there is a medical concern. Some medical issues require more frequent monitoring than every 2 years.

Q: If a driver fails a DOT exam but still holds a prior medical card that has not expired, can he or she drive a CMV?
A: No. Once a new medical exam is completed (and is not in "pending" status), the results of that exam take precedence over any previous exams. That is, if a driver fails an exam but still holds an unexpired medical card from a previous exam, that card is no longer valid.

OVERVIEW

Responsibility for Compliance

Compliance with the medical qualification standards is
a shared responsibility:

Party	Responsibility
Drivers	• Must not drive a CMV unless medically qualified.
	• Must not drive a CMV if too ill or fatigued to drive safely.
	• Must carry proof of medical certification unless such proof is contained in the driver's CDL driving record.
	• Must carry proof of any medical variance.
	• For CDL drivers: must provide all necessary documentation to state driver licensing agency concerning medical certification.
	• Must obtain DOT exams from examiners who are listed on the National Registry of Certified Medical Examiners.
Motor carriers	• Must not allow a driver to drive a CMV unless he/she is medically qualified and is not too ill or fatigued to drive safely.
	• Must maintain all required documentation of each driver's medical certification.
	• Must ensure that current medical forms and certificates are being used.
	• Must ensure that chosen medical examiners are qualified to perform DOT medical exams.
	• Must ensure that medical exams are being performed by examiners who are listed on the National Registry of Certified Medical Examiners.

Party	Responsibility
Medical examiners	• Must be knowledgeable of the physical and mental demands placed on CMV drivers. • Must be knowledgeable of the DOT medical standards, including the Medical Advisory Criteria. • Must be proficient in using the medical protocols necessary to adequately perform DOT medical exams. • Must be listed on the National Registry of Certified Medical Examiners if performing DOT exams for interstate CMV drivers. • Must use current DOT medical exam forms and certificates.

Q: Who has to pay for DOT medical exams?
A: The FMCSA does not address the issue of payment for medical exams. That issue is left for employers, drivers, and labor organizations to decide, in compliance with state labor laws.

Q: Our driver's medical card is still valid but he/she developed a medical condition that could affect safe driving. Should the driver be sent for a new exam?
A: Yes. The driver *must* be sent for a new DOT exam if the driver or company determines that the driver may be unsafe to drive, even if the current medical card is valid.

OVERVIEW

25

Who Can Perform a DOT Medical Exam?

A healthcare provider is authorized to perform a DOT medical
exam for an interstate driver only
if he or she is listed on the National Registry of Certified Medical Examiners. The Registry is
available online at:

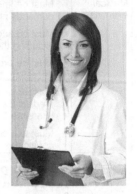

nationalregistry.fmcsa.dot.gov

The motor carrier must perform
the following steps before allowing a driver to operate a CMV in
interstate commerce:

1. Verify that the driver was certified by a medical examiner who was listed on the Registry on the date
   the certificate was issued.

2. Place documentation of that fact in the driver's
   qualification file. This "note" or other documentation can be removed from the file three years after
   its creation.

Key points:

- If an examiner who is listed on the Registry is later
  removed from the Registry, the medical certificates
  that that examiner issued do not become invalidated;
  they will remain valid until they expire.

- There are no exceptions based on how far away the
  nearest Registry-listed examiner is located from the
  driver. In some cases, drivers may need to travel to
  find a qualified examiner.

- The medical exam certificate contains a space for the
  examiner's National Registry Number. This space
  must be completed after any DOT exam performed
  on an interstate driver. The ID number can be
  searched on the Registry website, to locate and verify
  the credentials of the examiner.

> DOT exams performed by someone who is <u>not</u> listed on the Registry will not be valid for interstate operations. State requirements may vary for intrastate-only drivers, however. Some states may choose NOT to require examiners to be listed on the Registry if performing exams on intrastate-only drivers. Motor carriers involved in intrastate commerce should check with their state to determine if their examiners must be listed on the National Registry.

To be considered qualified, a medical examiner must also:

• Know the specific physical and mental demands of driving a commercial motor vehicle;

• Know the federal medical requirements (49 CFR Part 391, Subpart E);

• Know the Medical Advisory Criteria (Appendix A to Part 391); and

• Be proficient in the use of — and actually use — the medical protocols needed to adequately perform the medical exam.

> A licensed optometrist can (but is not required to) perform the visual portion of the exam.

To be listed on the Registry, an examiner must:

• Be licensed, certified, or registered under state laws and regulations to perform physical exams (this can include, for example, medical doctors, osteopaths, physician assistants, advanced practice nurses, and chiropractors);

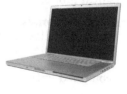

• Log onto the Registry website and receive a unique identifier;

• Complete required training;

• Pass a certification test;

- Submit to periodic monitoring and audits; and

- Maintain their certification by completing periodic training every 5 years and passing the certification exam every 10 years.

An alternative process for getting onto the Registry exists for medical examiners who work for the Department of Veterans Affairs (VA). These examiners may only perform driver medical exams for veterans enrolled in the VA healthcare system.

Examiners are required to report results of driver exams to the FMCSA by midnight (local time) of the next calendar day via the National Registry system.

Regulations, Guidelines, and Standards

The Federal Motor Carrier Safety Regulations include 13 broad medical standards to be met by all commercial motor vehicle drivers. Examiners, however, must be familiar with much more than the regulations alone. The FMCSA has also issued a variety of medical guidelines, interpretations, recommendations, and criteria to be considered.

Those charged with reviewing a driver's physical qualifications need to distinguish between the federal medical standards (as found in 49 CFR §391.41) and federal medical guidelines:

- **Regulations/standards** are mandates that (by law) must be followed. For example, the physical qualification regulations for CMV drivers involved in interstate commerce are found in §391.41(b) and must be complied with.

- **Guidelines,** such as the Medical Advisory Criteria and medical conference reports, are recommendations, not law. Guidelines are intended as "best practices" only.

Guidelines have been issued by the FMCSA to provide additional information and are based on medical literature. If an examiner chooses not to follow the guidelines, the FMCSA says the reason(s) for the variation should be documented. However, the examiner is ultimately responsible for determining if a CMV driver is medically qualified and is safe to drive under the regulations.

Non-regulatory medical standards change more frequently than the regulations do. Therefore, a medical examiner may make changes to his or her standards for qualifying a driver even though the regulations have not changed, as long as those standards comply with current regulations.

Regulations

The FMCSA administers the following regulations pertaining to the DOT medical exam, many of which can be found in Chapter 9. Note that – unlike guidelines and recommendations – regulations cannot normally be changed without the FMCSA first providing notice to the public and offering an opportunity for the public to comment on the change.

Regulation	Description
§391.11	Describes the minimum driver qualification standards, including the need to be at least 21 years old and be physically qualified to drive.
§391.41	Describes the physical qualification requirements for drivers, including 13 standards used to determine whether drivers are medically fit for duty. Four of the standards are not open to clinical interpretation: vision, hearing, epilepsy, and diabetes mellitus (but see §391.46). The other nine are discretionary standards, open to clinical judgment.
§391.43	Describes the responsibilities of the medical examiner, including instructions for performing the medical exam, a description of driver tasks and work environment, the sample Medical Examination Report form, and the Medical Examiner's Certificate.
§391.44	Describes the alternate vision standard and procedures by which a driver can become medically certified.
§391.45	Identifies who must be examined, and when.

OVERVIEW

29

Regulation	Description
§391.46	Describes the procedures that insulin-treated diabetic drivers must use to become medically certified.
§391.47	Describes the process for conflict resolution when there is a disagreement between the driver's primary care provider and the medical examiner for the motor carrier concerning driver qualifications.
§391.49	Describes the Skill Performance Evaluation (SPE) Certification Program, which is an alternative qualification standard for drivers with limb disorders who cannot physically qualify to drive under §391.41(b)(1) or (b)(2). NOTE: The SPE program was created in 1964 and was known as the Handicapped Driver Waiver Program.
§391.62	Describes limited exemptions for intra-city zone drivers.
§391.64	Describes grandfathering for certain drivers who participated in vision and diabetes waiver study programs. These drivers may be certified as long as they continue to meet the provisions outlined in §391.64 and continue to meet all other qualification standards. (**NOTE:** The diabetes waiver study program was withdrawn effective November 19, 2019.)
Part 391, Appendix A	Contains the Medical Advisory Criteria, which are advisory guidelines for medical examiners.
Part 390	Includes general information and definitions (§390.5), as well as the requirements for medical examiners to get listed on (or removed from) the National Registry.
Part 40	Describes DOT procedures for drug and alcohol testing.

The Two Absolutes

The federal regulations in §391.41 include 13 specific standards that drivers must meet in order to be considered qualified to drive a CMV. While the medical examiner can use his or her discretion when judging a driver on most of those 13 criteria, two of the standards are considered "absolutes." That is, the examiner is not given leeway to certify a driver who doesn't meet one or more of those two standards.

Drivers with insulin-controlled diabetes may qualify under §391.46 and drivers who do not meet the vision standard may in both eyes may qualify under the alternate vision standard in §391.44.

The two "absolutes" are the standards for:

• Hearing

• Epilepsy

Just because a driver fails one of the medical standards does not mean that that individual can never be medically certified to drive. The driver could take one of several paths to get back behind the wheel. He or she could:

• **Apply for an exemption from the FMCSA.** The agency issues temporary exemptions from the hearing and epilepsy standards. An exemption allows a driver to operate a CMV in interstate commerce despite having a disqualifying medical condition. The FMCSA has applications and/or more information about these exemptions on their Medical Programs website. Exemptions are regulated under 49 CFR Part 381. Questions can be directed to the FMCSA at (703) 448-3094 or by e-mail to medicalexemptions@dot.gov.

• **Follow the procedures in §391.44 if not qualfied under the vision standard in 391.41(b)(10).** A driver who does not meet the vision standard in both eyes, may be certified for up to one year by following the procedures in §391.44 if qualified based on the vision in the better eye. This involves an optometrist/ opthalmologist completing a Vision Evaluation Report (MCSA-5871) no more than 45 days prior to the DOT exam for the driver to present to the DOT medical examiner. The certified medical examiner then makes the certification decision.

• **Follow the procedures in §391.46 if using insulin.** A driver with insulin-treated diabetes mellitus may be certified for up to one year by following the procedures in §391.46. This involves providing his/ her treating clinician with blood glucose self-monitoring records and providing a completed MCSA-5870 form to his/her DOT medical exam, who then makes the certification decision.

OVERVIEW

31

- **Apply for an exemption from the state.** Many states offer exemption programs to drivers who wish to be engaged in intrastate (in-state-only) commerce. Drivers should check with their state enforcement or licensing agency for details.

- **Wait until the condition improves.** Though not always possible, drivers with a disqualifying medical condition may be medically certified in the future if the condition improves.

Medical Advisory Criteria

The FMCSA provides a list of "Medical Advisory Criteria" to help examiners evaluate driver fitness. These guidelines are based on expert review and are considered "best practices."

Medical examiners can choose to follow or ignore the guidelines because they are not regulations. However, when an examiner makes a certification decision that does not conform with the FMCSA's guidelines or recommendations, the examiner should document why the guidelines were not followed.

The Medical Advisory Criteria can be found in Appendix A to Part 391, found in Chapter 9.

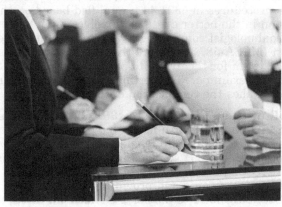

Medical Expert Panel Reports

Reports from the FMCSA's Medical Expert Panel (MEP) provide insight and recommendations concerning medical conditions affecting driver qualification. The MEP is an independent panel of physicians, clinicians, and scientists who are experts in their field. The MEP reviews relevant research and submits its opinions to the FMCSA on the driver qualification standards. The MEP has no authority to change the regulations, however.

The FMCSA provides two types of reports for each medical condition examined. The first is an "evidence" report, a systematic review of research on specific questions regarding medical conditions and driving. The second is the report from the MEP itself, with opinions and recommendations aimed at the FMCSA.

The MEP reports are available on the FMCSA and/or the National Transportation Library websites (see Chapter 9 for links).

Among the MEP report topics available:

- Traumatic brain injury
- Diabetes mellitus
- Schedule II medications
- Cardiovascular disease
- Seizure disorders
- Sleep disorders
- Renal disease
- Vision
- Musculoskeletal disease
- Hearing
- Psychiatric disease
- Stroke

OVERVIEW

- Multiple sclerosis and Parkinson's disease

- Substance abuse

Medical Conference/Advisory Reports

Over the years, the FMCSA has gathered a variety of medical conference reports and advisory panel reports relating to specific medical conditions. Some of these reports are referenced in the Medical Advisory Criteria (as found on the Medical Examination Report form and elsewhere), and many are superseded by the Medical Expert Panel reports described above. Select reports (dating back to 1988) are available on the FMCSA website.

State Regulations for In-State-Only Drivers

The federal medical regulations and standards described above and throughout this guide apply to drivers and motor carriers engaged in interstate commerce. Drivers involved in *intrastate* commerce may or may not have to follow the same rules.

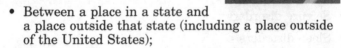

Interstate commerce is trade, traffic, or transportation in the United States:

- Between a place in a state and a place outside that state (including a place outside of the United States);

- Between two places in a state through another state or a place outside of the United States; or

- Between two places in a state as part of trade, traffic, or transportation originating or terminating outside the state or the United States.

Note that a vehicle does not need to cross state lines in order for the transportation to be considered "interstate" commerce!

Commerce conducted entirely within a single state and not considered "interstate" commerce is "*intra*state" commerce and falls beyond the jurisdiction of the FMCSA. However, the FMCSA can refuse to provide highway funds to a state whose regulations are not substantially similar to the federal standards. Thus, most states choose to make their laws similar or identical to the federal standards.

Section 350.341 specifies what "substantially similar" means:

- States may exempt drivers of vehicles that weigh less than 26,001 pounds, as long as they are not hauling hazardous materials requiring placards.

- States can have "grandfather" clauses. They can exempt drivers from the federal physical qualification standards if three conditions are met:

  1. The driver was qualified under existing state laws at the time the state adopted qualification standards compatible with the federal standards;

  2. The otherwise non-qualifying medical or physical condition has not substantially worsened; and

  3. No other non-qualifying medical or physical condition has developed.

- States may issue variances to intrastate drivers with medical or physical conditions that would otherwise be non-qualifying, if those variances are based on sound medical judgment and do not harm highway safety.

- States may decide not to adopt a "registry" of qualified medical examiners, such as (or similar to) the National Registry of Certified Medical Examiners.

Drivers involved in intrastate commerce are subject to the state's laws and regulations. In most cases, the state rules mirror the federal rules, but there are exceptions. In some cases, the state rules are less restrictive

OVERVIEW

35

or may not apply to the same types of vehicles as the federal rules. Drivers who are unqualified to drive in interstate commerce may be able to drive in intrastate commerce by applying for a waiver or exemption.

Consult your state laws and regulations for details.

Company Standards

Motor carriers have some discretion to set their own standards for medical qualifica-
tion, above and beyond state or federal standards. Section 390.3(d) gives employers the right to adopt stricter medical standards; less-restrictive standards are not allowed. In addition, em-
ployers can require drivers to be physically able to perform non-
driving duties as a condition of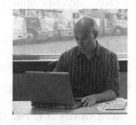
employment, although those company standards are not applied during the medical exam.

> The medical examiner does not apply company standards during a DOT medical exam, even if the company is paying for the exam. In other words, the examiner may certify a driver even if that driver does not meet the employer's standards.

Careful consideration must be given to any company-specific, medical-related standards! If they are job related and consistent with business necessity, they may be acceptable. If not, they run the risk of violating the *Americans with Disabilities Act*.

III. The Job of Commercial Driving

Note: J. J. Keller & Associates, Inc. grants permission to purchasers of this Guide to reproduce this chapter for use by their medical examiners, provided that J. J. Keller's copyright remains visible on all copies.

The Driver and Their Role

Commercial motor vehicle (CMV) drivers come in all shapes and sizes, not to mention ages, sexes, ethnicities, creeds, and colors. But a common denominator among all drivers is that they must all meet the same basic standards for physical, mental, and emotional health.

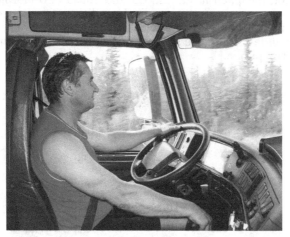

The medical examiner is charged with making sure those standards are met. Together with motor carriers, they help ensure safety on the nation's highways by keeping physically and mentally unqualified individuals from getting behind the wheel.

Therefore, motor carriers and – especially – medical examiners must be aware of the rigorous physical, mental, and emotional demands placed on CMV drivers. In the interest of public safety:

- The medical examiner is required to certify that the driver does not have any physical, mental, or organic condition that might affect the driver's ability to operate a CMV safely.

- The motor carrier is required to ensure that the driver remains qualified to drive and is re-examined when conditions warrant.

The CMV driver population has characteristics similar to the general population – including all its ills, like obesity and aging. An aging workforce means a higher risk exists for chronic diseases, deficiencies, gradual or sudden incapacitation, and the likelihood of comorbidity (two or more coexisting medical conditions or diseases). All of these can interfere with the ability to drive safely, thus endangering the safety and health of the driver and the public.

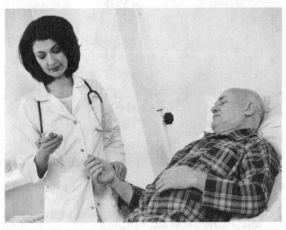

According to the Federal Motor Carrier Safety Administration (FMCSA), the average truck or bus driver is:

- Male,
- More than 40 years old,
- Sedentary,
- Overweight,
- A smoker, and
- Has poor eating habits.

The typical CMV driver also:

- Is less healthy than the average person,
- Has more than two medical conditions, and
- Is more likely to have cardiovascular disease.

Stress Factors

Many factors contribute to making commercial driving a stressful occupation:

Types of Routes

- Turn-around or short-relay routes allow the driver to return home each evening.

- A long-relay route requires driving 9 to 11 hours, followed by at least a 10-hour off-duty period. Several days may elapse before the driver returns home.

- With a straight-through-haul or cross-country route, the driver may spend a month on the road, dispatched from one load to the next. The driver usually sleeps in the truck and returns home for only four or five days before leaving for another extended period on the road.

- In a team operation, drivers share the driving by alternating their driving and rest periods.

CMV DRIVING

III. The Job of Commercial Driving

Schedules

- Abrupt schedule changes and rotating work schedules may result in irregular sleep patterns and a driver beginning a trip already fatigued.

- Tight pickup and delivery schedules require both day and night driving. Failure to meet schedules may result in a financial loss for the driver.

- Long hours and extended time away from family and friends may result in a lack of social support.

Environment

- The driver may be exposed to excessive vehicle noise, vibration, diesel exhaust, and extremes in temperature.

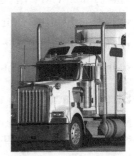

- The driver may encounter adverse road, weather, and traffic conditions that cause unavoidable delays.

Types of Cargo

- The driver of a bus is responsible for passenger safety. Transporting passengers also demands effective social skills.

- Loss or shifting of cargo while driving can result in serious accidents.

- Transporting hazardous materials, including explosives, flammables, and toxics, increases the risk of injury and property damage extending beyond the accident site.

Driving and Other Tasks

The following are some of the most common tasks that drivers must be able to perform as part of their career.

Medical examiners and carriers must be aware of the demands placed on drivers when performing these tasks.

Staying Alert When Driving

- Being vigilant and attentive while driving demands sustained mental alertness and physical endurance, without being compromised by fatigue or sudden, incapacitating symptoms.

- Drivers need cognitive skills like problem solving, communication, judgment, and appropriate behavior in both normal and emergency situations.

- Driving requires the ability to judge the appropriate speed under changing traffic, road, and weather conditions.

Using Side Mirrors

- Mirrors on both sides of the vehicle are used to monitor traffic that can move into the driver's blind spot.

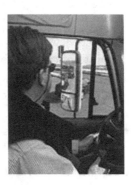

- Mirrors are also used in backing up vehicles to loading and unloading areas. Sufficient lateral cervical mobility is needed for effective use of side mirrors.

Controlling a Steering Wheel

- Steering wheels of large trucks and buses are oversized.

- The act of steering can be simulated by offering resistance while having the driver imitate the motion pattern necessary to turn a 24-inch steering wheel.

Manipulating Dashboard Switches and Controls

- Large trucks and buses are complex vehicles with multiple dashboards, switches, and knobs.

- Use of these components requires adequate reach, prehension (the ability to grasp firmly), and touch sensation in hands and fingers.

Shifting Gears

- The manual transmission of a large truck may have more than 20 gears.

- Shifting requires the driver to repeatedly perform reciprocal movements of both legs coordinated with right arm and hand movements.

Entering and Exiting the Vehicle

- The driver may have to enter and exit the vehicle similar to the way an individual climbs a ladder, by maintaining three points of contact for safety.

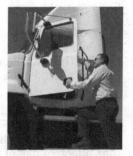

- Full overhead extension may be required to reach the hand-holds.

- Hip angle and knee flexion may both have to exceed 90°.

Coupling and Uncoupling Trailers

- Multiple sub-tasks are performed in the process of coupling and uncoupling trailers, including raising and lowering the trailer supports, connecting air lines and electrical cables, and checking the height of the trailer kingpin.

- Physical demands include grip strength, upper body strength, range of motion, balance, and flexibility.

Loading, Securing, and Unloading Cargo

- FMCSA guidelines do not specify the number of pounds a driver must be able to lift.

- Loading and unloading a truck and standing while lifting heavy objects of 50 pounds or more are typical, and they require the individual to exert greater than 6.0 metabolic equivalents (MET) (more than 7 kcal/min), similar to heavy construction work, firefighting, or coal mining. A six-MET activity requires six times the metabolic energy needed for sitting quietly.

Performing Vehicle Checks

- Grip strength, upper- and lower-body strength, range of motion, balance, and flexibility are required to inspect the engine, brakes, and cargo.

- Vision and hearing are used to identify and interpret changes in vehicle performance.

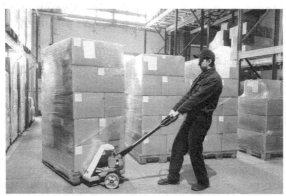

IV. The Medical Exam

Fitness for Duty

The periodic physical examination required of most commercial motor vehicle (CMV) drivers is described as a "medical fitness for duty" exam. Its purpose is to detect the presence of any physical, mental, or organic conditions that could affect the ability of the driver to operate a CMV safely.

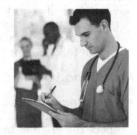

Under FMCSA regulations, 49 CFR §391.43, *Medical examination; certificate of physical qualification*, describes the medical examiner's responsibilities: to determine medical fitness for duty and issue Medical Examiner's Certificates to CMV drivers who meet the physical qualification standards.

According to the FMCSA, a medical examiner's "fundamental obligation" is "to establish whether a driver has a disease, disorder, or injury resulting in a higher than acceptable likelihood for gradual or sudden incapacitation or sudden death, thus endangering public safety."

Risk

Risk is the probability that an event will occur within a certain period of time. Determining "acceptable risk" is both a medical and societal decision.

Medical examiners need to ask themselves, "Does the driver pose a risk to public safety?" Any time they answer "yes," they should not certify the driver as medically fit for duty.

Considering Safety

During a DOT physical exam, the examiner must consider:

Physical Condition

- Symptoms — Does a benign underlying condition with an excellent prognosis have symptoms that interfere with driving ability (for example, a benign arrhythmia that causes fainting)?

- Incapacitation — Is the onset of incapacitating symptoms so *rapid* that they interfere with safe driving, or can the driver stop the vehicle safely before becoming incapacitated? On the other hand, is the onset so *gradual* that the driver is unaware of their effect?

Mental Condition

- Cognitive — Can the driver process environmental cues rapidly and make appropriate responses, independently solve problems, and function in a changing environment?

- Behavior — Are the driver's interactions with other people appropriate, responsible, and nonviolent?

Medical Treatment

- Effects — Does treatment allow the driver to perform tasks safer than without treatment?

- Side effects — Do side effects interfere with safe driving (e.g., drowsiness, dizziness, blurred vision, or changes in mental status)?

THE EXAM

Medical Examiner's Obligations

The medical examiner's role is making sure the driver is medically fit for duty, not diagnosing and treating personal medical conditions. Nonetheless, the examiner has a responsibility to educate and refer the driver for further evaluation if he/she suspects an undiagnosed or worsening medical problem. The examiner should:

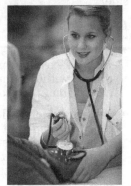

- Comply with FMCSA regulations;

- Seek further testing/evaluation for medical conditions about which the examiner is unsure;

- Refer the driver to his/her personal healthcare provider for diagnosis and treatment of potential medical conditions discovered during the exam; and

- Promote public safety by educating the driver about:

  - Side effects caused by the use of prescription and/or over-the-counter medications;

  - Medication warning labels and how to read them; and

  - The importance of seeking appropriate intervention for non-disqualifying conditions, especially those that, if neglected, could result in serious illness and possible future disqualification.

Medical Examination Report Form

DOT medical examiners need to perform driver physical exams and record the findings according to the instructions on the FMCSA's Medical Examination Report Form (MCSA-5875), as shown in §391.43 (see also Chapter 5). Whether a driver can be certified depends on whether he or she meets the requirements of the FMCSA's physical qualification standards in §391.41.

The following is an overview of how the exam form is to be completed, including its organization, required signatures, and minimum documentation.

Medical Record Number

The form begins with a space to record a Medical Record number. This field is optional, but may be used to tie the exam form to the driver's medical record by entering the corresponding record number.

> **MEDICAL RECORD #**
>
> 7654321
>
> *(or sticker)*

Section 1: Driver Information

The driver completes Section 1 (except the entry for "Driver ID Verified By"), but the medical examiner is expected to review the information the driver entered to be sure it's legible and complete. The following is a description of each required item and what to look for:

PERSONAL INFORMATION

- **Driver Name (last, first, middle initial)** — Verify that the order is correct, with last name first.

- **Date of Birth** — Verify the month, day, and year.

- **Age** — Verify that the date of birth agrees with the age given.

- **Address** — The driver's current address.

- **Driver's License Number** — Taken from the driver's license to drive. This does not necessarily need to be a commercial driver's license (CDL). The motor carrier is responsible for ensuring that the driver has the proper license for the equipment to be operated.

- **Issuing State/Province** — The state or Canadian province that issued the driver's license. The two-letter postal abbreviation is adequate

- **Phone and E-mail** — Verify area code and current home or cell phone number. E-mail is optional.

- **CLP/CDL Applicant/Holder** — If yes, verify that the driver has or will be applying for a CDL or commercial learner's permit (CLP).

> NOTE: The rules do not include an application deadline. Therefore, examiners are not required to verify if and when drivers who checked "Yes" will be applying for a CDL or CLP.

- **Driver ID Verified By** — This item is completed by the medical examiner or staff, to note the *type of photo ID* used to verify the driver's identity, such as CDL, driver's license, passport, etc.

- **Has your USDOT/FMCSA medical certificate ever been denied or issued for less than two years?** — Verify a selection. A "yes" response should result in further questioning.

? **Q: Can a DOT exam be performed on a driver who is under 21 years old, who doesn't speak English, or who otherwise is unqualified to drive?**
A: Yes. The motor carrier is responsible for ensuring that the driver meets the qualification requirements (such as being at least 21 years old) before driving a CMV involved in interstate commerce. The medical examiner can administer a DOT physical exam to anyone who requests the exam, even those who may be otherwise unqualified to drive.

Health History

The purpose of the health history is to obtain information that could help detect conditions that could affect safe driving. Providing false information on the health history can result in fines and penalties.

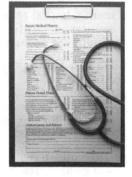

The medical examiner is expected to review the information to make sure it's legible and complete. The examiner also must discuss with the driver any "yes" or "not sure" answers, as well as potential hazards of using medications while driving, including herbal, diet, and over-the-counter medications. This discussion must then be documented on the form in Section 2.

DRIVER HEALTH HISTORY

| Have you ever had surgery? If "yes," please list and explain below. | ⊗ Yes ○ No ○ Not Sure |

Hernia repaired in 1997 — right side, inguinal

| Are you currently taking medications (prescription, over-the-counter, herbal remedies, diet supplements)? If "yes," please describe below. | ⊗ Yes ○ No ○ Not Sure |

Daily multi-vitamin

(Attach additional sheets if necessary)

- **Have you ever had surgery?** — If yes, the driver should include as many details as possible, i.e., types of surgeries, dates, etc. This question is deliberately open-ended, with no limits on the types of surgeries to include. It's up to the examiner to decide if any past surgery might have a current effect on safety.

- **Are you currently taking medications?** — The driver should check "yes" if taking any diet supplements, herbal remedies, or prescription or over-the-counter medications of any type. If yes, the driver should list the name(s) and dosage(s).

- **Health History (page 2)** — The driver must check either the "Yes," "No," or "Not Sure" box for each of the 32 items listed, to indicate whether the driver ever had the listed symptom or condition. Space is provided for any additional health conditions not listed.

- **Did you answer "yes" to any of questions 1-32?** — For any "Yes" response on the medical history, verify that the driver has provided additional information, which could include onset date, diagnosis, medications, limitations resulting from the condition, contact information for the treating healthcare provider, etc.

DRIVER HEALTH HISTORY *(continued)*

Do you have or have you ever had:	Yes	No	Not Sure		Yes	No	Not Sure
1. Head/brain injuries or illnesses (e.g., concussion)	O	⊗	O	16. Dizziness, headaches, numbness, tingling, or memory loss	O	⊗	O
2. Seizures, epilepsy	O	⊗	O	17. Unexplained weight loss	O	⊗	O
3. Eye problems (except glasses or contacts)	O	⊗	O	18. Stroke, mini-stroke (TIA), paralysis, or weakness	O	⊗	O
4. Ear and/or hearing problems	O	⊗	O	19. Missing or limited use of arm, hand, finger, leg, foot, toe	O	⊗	O
5. Heart disease, heart attack, bypass, or other heart problems	O	⊗	O	20. Neck or back problems	O	⊗	O
6. Pacemaker, stents, implantable devices, or other heart procedures	O	⊗	O	21. Bone, muscle, joint, or nerve problems	O	⊗	O
7. High blood pressure	O	⊗	O	22. Blood clots or bleeding problems	O	⊗	O
8. High cholesterol	O	⊗	O	23. Cancer	O	⊗	O
9. Chronic (long-term) cough, shortness of breath, or other breathing problems	O	⊗	O	24. Chronic (long-term) infection or other chronic diseases	O	⊗	O
10. Lung disease (e.g., asthma)	O	⊗	O	25. Sleep disorders, pauses in breathing while asleep, daytime sleepiness, loud snoring	⊗	O	O
11. Kidney problems, kidney stones, or pain/problems with urination	O	⊗	O	26. Have you ever had a sleep test (e.g., sleep apnea)?	O	⊗	O
12. Stomach, liver, or digestive problems	⊗	O	O	27. Have you ever spent a night in the hospital?	O	⊗	O
13. Diabetes or blood sugar problems	O	⊗	O	28. Have you ever had a broken bone?	O	⊗	O
Insulin used	O	⊗	O	29. Have you ever used or do you now use tobacco?	O	⊗	O
14. Anxiety, depression, nervousness, other mental health problems	O	⊗	O	30. Do you currently drink alcohol?	O	⊗	O
				31. Have you used an illegal substance within the past two years?	O	⊗	O
15. Fainting or passing out	O	⊗	O	32. Have you ever failed a drug test or been dependent on an illegal substance?	O	⊗	O

Other health condition(s) not described above: ○Yes ⊗No ○ Not Sure

Did you answer "yes" to any of questions 1-32? If so, please comment further on those health conditions below. ⊗Yes ○No ○ Not Sure

Some acid reflux. 2-3 times/month. Wife says I snore.

- **CMV Driver's Signature** — Through the signature, the driver is:

  - Certifying that all the information he/she entered is "accurate and complete," and

  - Acknowledging that providing inaccurate or false information or omitting information could invalidate the exam and certificate and result in a civil or criminal penalty against the driver.

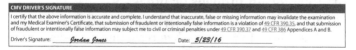

CMV DRIVER'S SIGNATURE

I certify that the above information is accurate and complete. I understand that inaccurate, false or missing information may invalidate the examination and my Medical Examiner's Certificate, that submission of fraudulent or intentionally false information is a violation of 49 CFR 390.35, and that submission of fraudulent or intentionally false information may subject me to civil or criminal penalties under 49 CFR 390.37 and 49 CFR 386 Appendices A and B.

Driver's Signature: *Jordan Jones*   Date: **5/23/16**

Section 2. Examination Report

The medical examiner completes the remainder of the form, beginning with a review of the driver's health history. The examiner is required to complete the entire medical exam even if he/she detects a medical condition that is considered disqualifying, such as deafness.

51

Medical Examiner's Obligations

The medical examiner is expected to review the driver's health history and discuss any "yes" or "not sure" responses. For each "yes" on the health history, the examiner should:

- Ask the driver about the condition's history, diagnosis, treatment, and response to treatment.

- Explore the underlying cause, precipitating events, and other relevant facts.

- Order additional tests or consultations as necessary to assess the driver's medical fitness.

- Review and discuss driver response to treatment and medications currently or recently used, including over-the-counter medications, and discuss any potential effects and side effects that may interfere with driving. As needed, the examiner may also educate the driver regarding drug interactions with other prescription and non-prescription drugs and alcohol.

- Write all information on the Medical Examination Report form.

> Of course, the examiner can ask other questions to help gather enough information to make the qualification decision.

Guidance for Analyzing a Driver's Health History

❏ Head/brain injuries or illnesses

A "Yes" response should prompt questions that help determine if the driver has recurring episodes of illness or any lasting physical, cognitive, or behavioral effects that interfere with the ability to drive safely.

❏ **Seizures, epilepsy**

A "Yes" response should prompt questions to decide whether the driver has a diagnosis of epilepsy (two or more unprovoked seizures), or whether the driver has had one seizure. The examiner should also gather information about type of seizure, duration, frequency of seizure activity, and date of last seizure.

NOTE: According to regulation, a driver with an established medical history or clinical diagnosis of epilepsy does not meet qualification standards and cannot be certified.

❏ **Eye problems**

The examiner should ask about changes in vision, diagnoses of eye disorders, and diagnoses commonly associated with secondary eye changes that interfere with driving. Complaints of glare or near-crashes may be the first warning signs of an eye disorder that interferes with safe driving. **Note:** If the driver does not meet the vision standard in both eyes, the driver may qualify under the alternate vision standard in §391.44 if they provide a Vision Evaluation Report (MCSA-5871) from an optometrist/opthalmologist dated 45 days or less prior to the date of the exam.

❏ **Ear and/or hearing problems**

The driver should be asked about changes in hearing, ringing in the ears, difficulties with balance, or dizziness. Loss of balance while performing non-driving tasks can lead to serious injury.

❏ **Heart disease, heart attack, bypass, or other heart problems**

The driver should be asked about history and symptoms of cardiovascular disease (CVD), syncope, dyspnea, congestive heart failure, angina, etc.

THE EXAM

NOTE: If the driver reports symptoms consistent with undiagnosed CVD, the driver should be referred to a specialist for further evaluation prior to certification. If a driver reports current CVD, the examiner should consult with the driver's health-care provider and obtain documentation prior to certification.

❏ **Pacemaker, stents, implantable devices, or other heart procedures**

The examiner should ask about any history of heart surgery, bypass, valve replacement, pacemaker, or angioplasty, and whether the driver has an implantable cardioverter defibrillator (ICD). The examiner may need to obtain heart-surgery information – including such things as copies of the original cardiac catheterization report, stress tests, worksheets, and original tracings – as needed to adequately assess the driver.

NOTE: If a driver gives a "Yes" answer to the question regarding heart procedures, the examiner is expected to obtain documentation from the cardiologist before certifying. Also, FMCSA medical guidelines recommend to not certify a driver who has an ICD, due to the risk of fainting and/or gradual or sudden incapacitation while driving a CMV. This includes a dual pacemaker/ICD, even if the ICD has not been activated.

❏ **High blood pressure**

The driver should be asked about his/her history, diagnosis, and treatment of hypertension, including his/her response to prescribed medications.

Hypertension alone is unlikely to cause sudden collapse. The likelihood increases, however, when there is target organ damage, particularly cerebral vascular disease. Recommending specific therapy is beyond the scope of the physical exam. The medical examiner, however, should be concerned with the blood pressure response to treatment, and whether the driver is free of any effects or side effects that could impair job performance.

❏ **Chronic (long-term) cough, shortness of breath, or other breathing problems**

Drivers suffering from shortness of breath should be asked what activities precipitate the episodes, and about the nature and characteristics of the episodes.

NOTE: According to guidelines, many drivers may experience shortness of breath while performing the non-driving aspects of their work (e.g., loading and unloading, etc.). However, most commercial drivers are not short of breath while driving their vehicles. Shortness of breath while driving should trigger a more detailed evaluation that can include consulting with a medical specialist.

❏ **Lung disease**

A "Yes" response should prompt questions about emergency room visits, hospitalizations, supplemental use of oxygen, use of inhalers and other medications, risk of exposure to allergens, etc.

NOTE: Since a driver must be alert at all times, any change in mental state is in direct conflict with highway safety. Even the slightest impairment in respiratory function under emergency conditions (when greater oxygen supply is necessary for performance) may be detrimental to safe driving.

❏ **Kidney problems, kidney stones, or pain/ problems with urination**

The driver should be asked about the degree and stability of renal impairment, ability to maintain treatment schedules, and the presence and status of any co-existing diseases.

THE EXAM

NOTE: If the driver is on dialysis, he/she cannot drive.

❏ **Stomach, liver, or digestive problems**

Drivers with stomach, liver, or digestive problems should be asked about the condition's history, diagnosis, treatment, and response to treatment and medications. The examiner is expected to explore the underlying cause, precipitating events, and other pertinent facts, and obtain additional tests or consultations as necessary.

❏ **Diabetes or blood sugar problems**

A "Yes" response should prompt questions about treatment, whether by diet, oral medications, Byetta, or insulin.

NOTE: Drivers with insulin-treated diabetes mellitus who are otherwise qualified may be certified for up to one year if they provide the examiner with a completed MCSA-5870 form from their treating clinician and meet certain qualification standards as described in §391.46. There are no longer any federal waiver or exemption programs for insulin-using drivers. If the driver is certified, the medical examiner must check the box at the end of the form for "Meets standards but periodic monitoring required" and enter "insulin treatment."

❏ **Anxiety, depression, nervousness, other mental health problems**

The examiner should ask the driver about the condition's history, diagnosis, treatment, and response to treatment and medications; explore underlying cause, precipitating events, and other pertinent facts; and obtain additional tests or consultations as necessary.

❑ **Fainting or passing out**

Drivers who check "Yes" should be asked whether they did so due to fainting or due to dizziness. They should also be asked about the episode(s), including frequency, factors leading to and surrounding an episode, and any associated neurologic symptoms (e.g., headache, nausea, loss of consciousness, unusual skin sensations, etc.).

❑ **Stroke, mini-stroke (TIA), paralysis, or weakness**

The examiner should note any lasting paresthesia (unusual skin sensations), sensory deficit, or weakness as a result of stroke, and consider both time and risk for seizure.

❑ **Missing or limited use of arm, hand, finger, leg, foot, toe**

The examiner needs to determine whether the missing limb affects the ability to grasp or ability to perform normal tasks such as braking, clutching, accelerating, etc.

NOTE: Drivers can be exempt from this standard if they obtain a Skill Performance Evaluation (SPE) certificate. The certificate is designed for "fixed deficits" of the extremities (such as missing limbs) and cannot be used for progressive disorders.

❑ **Neck or back problems**

The examiner should ask about the degree of pain. How does the pain affect the ability of the driver to perform driving and non-driving tasks? What does the driver do to alleviate pain? Does the treatment interfere with safe driving?

❑ **Bone, muscle, joint, or nerve problems**

The examiner should ask the driver about history, diagnosis, and treatment of musculoskeletal conditions, such as rheumatic, arthritic, orthopedic, and

THE EXAM

57

IV. The Medical Exam

neuromuscular diseases. The diagnosis could indicate that the driver is at risk for sudden, incapacitating episodes of muscle weakness, loss of muscle control, skin sensations, low muscle tone, or pain. It could also indicate a degenerative process that over time will restrict movements and eventually interfere with the ability to safely operate a CMV.

NOTE: Musculoskeletal diseases may adversely impact the driver's muscle strength and agility needed to perform non-driving tasks such as coupling, uncoupling, loading, unloading, and inspecting the vehicle, lifting, installing tire chains, getting in and out of the cab, etc.

❏ **Sleep disorders, pauses in breathing while asleep, daytime sleepiness, loud snoring**

A "Yes" answer should lead to questions about sleep disorders and about such symptoms as daytime sleepiness, loud snoring, or pauses in breathing while asleep. When indicated, the examiner should screen for sleep disorders.

❏ **Do you currently drink alcohol?**

Drivers who frequently use alcohol should be asked about their consumption of alcohol, including quantity and frequency. The examiner may use tools such as the "CAGE" questionnaire to screen for possible alcohol-use problems. Drivers who show signs of a current alcoholic illness should be referred to a specialist.

Medical Examiner's Comments on Health History

At a minimum, the examiner's comments should include:

• The nature of any "Yes" or "Not Sure" responses on the health history and the effect on driving ability; and

• A discussion about medication and/or treatment effects and side effects that might interfere with driving ability.

SECTION 2. Examination Report *(to be filled out by the medical examiner)*

DRIVER HEALTH HISTORY REVIEW

Review and discuss pertinent driver answers and any available medical records. Comment on the driver's responses to the "health history" questions that may affect the driver's safe operation of a commercial motor vehicle (CMV).

Reports no daytime sleepiness. Recommended seeing PCP for diet and wt. management and evaluation of gastric upset.

(Attach additional sheets if necessary)

If the examiner obtains any supplementary medical reports to complete the health history, a copy of those reports should be filed with the medical exam form.

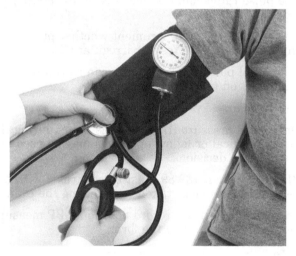

THE EXAM

Testing: Blood Pressure / Pulse Rate

The TESTING section of the exam form begins with a check of blood pressure and pulse rate and is to be completed by the medical examiner.

TESTING		
Pulse rate: ___76___ Pulse rhythm regular: ⊗ Yes ◯ No		
Blood Pressure	Systolic	Diastolic
Sitting	136	84
Second reading (optional)	132	81

The medical examiner must measure:

Pulse

- The pulse rate should be recorded in the space provided.

- The examiner should document whether pulse rhythm is regular ("Yes") or irregular ("No").

- Additional pulse characteristics can be recorded in comments on the form.

Blood Pressure

- Only blood pressure (BP) readings taken during the driver physical or follow-up exams may be used for certification decisions.

- BP greater than 139/89 must be confirmed with a second measurement taken later during the exam.

- The examiner should record additional BP measurements in comments on the form.

NOTE:

- The examiner must document his or her discussion with the driver about any history, medications, or abnormal findings related to hypertension.

- Trained assistants may take and record the BP and pulse.

- When BP, pulse rate, or both are significant factors in the examiner's decision not to certify a driver, the

FMCSA says it is "prudent" for the *examiner* to take the readings.

• No matter who takes the readings, the examiner must sign the form, thereby taking responsibility for and attesting to the validity of all documented test results.

The hypertension criteria are important because there is strong evidence that hypertension markedly increases the risk of cardiovascular disease and that effective treatment reduces cardiovascular morbidity and mortality. To be certified to drive, the driver should have ongoing hypertension management and be free of side effects that may impair safe driving.

Hypertension Guidelines

The Medical Advisory Criteria contain guidelines for certifying drivers based on their BP measurements over three stages of hypertension.

REMEMBER: These are *recommendations*. The medical examiner may use his/her clinical expertise and results of the individual driver exam to determine the length of time between recertification exams.

After confirming and recording a systolic reading of 140 or higher and/or a diastolic reading of 90 or higher, the first step is determining which stage of hypertension the driver has:

Reading	Category
140-159/90-99	Stage 1 hypertension
160-179/100-109	Stage 2 hypertension
greater than or equal to 180/110	Stage 3 hypertension

Q: What happens if the BP reading includes a systolic reading in one stage and a diastolic reading in a different stage?
A: The *higher* stage is used. For example, readings of 168/94 and 148/104 are both examples of Stage 2 hypertension.

IV. The Medical Exam

After determining the stage of hypertension, the examiner can refer to the recommendations for certifying or recertifying the driver, as follows:

Category	Expiration Date	Recertification
Stage 1	1 year	1 year if ≤140/90
Stage 2	One-time certificate for 3 months	1 year from date of exam if ≤140/90
Stage 3	6 months from date of examination if ≤140/90	6 months if ≤140/90

Stage 1 — A driver with Stage 1 hypertension may be certified for one year, giving the driver time to reduce BP to 140/90 or less. After that year, the driver should only be recertified annually, and only if BP remains at or below 140/90. However, if the driver has not achieved a BP less than or equal to 140/90 at recertification – and if BP is less than 160/100 – then a one-time, three-month certificate should be issued.

Stage 2 — A driver with Stage 2 hypertension may be certified one time for 3 months, to provide time to reduce BP to 140/90 or less. Anti-hypertensive drug therapy is recommended. After those 3 months, the driver should only be recertified annually, and only if BP remains at or below 140/90.

Stage 3 — A driver with Stage 3 hypertension may not be certified until he or she is able to reduce BP to 140/90 or less and treatment is well tolerated. Once BP falls below Stage 1, the driver may be certified for 6-month periods, as long as BP remains at or below 140/90.

A one-time, three-month med card is granted in two cases:
1. Where a driver has a BP that is equivalent to Stage 2 hypertension, or
2. Where a driver that was certified with Stage 1 hypertension has not achieved a BP less than or equal to 140/90 at recertification.

This three-month certificate is a one-time issuance for the recertification period and is not intended to mean once in the driver's lifetime.

Note that a driver with Stage 3 hypertension (greater than or equal to 180/110) is at an unacceptable risk for an acute hypertensive event and should be disqualified. The examiner can reconsider the driver for certification following effective treatment for hypertension, demonstrated by the driver's blood pressure being stabilized at less than or equal to 140/90.

➤ **If a driver with hypertension has lowered his/her blood pressure to normal range, lost weight, and is off medications, he/she <u>can</u> be certified for 2 years at the examiner's discretion.**

The 6-month expiration and recertification dates apply to a driver who:

- Has a known history of Stage 3 hypertension,

- Has an acceptable blood pressure at the time of the exam, and

- Tolerates treatment with no side effects affecting safe CMV operation.

? Q: Does the examiner need to repeat the whole exam for a BP re-check?
A: If the examiner completed an exam and issued a certificate to the driver, even for a short term, then the examiner must complete a new exam when the driver returns (e.g., 3 months later). The expiration date of any existing certificate cannot be extended. Once an exam is completed and a certification decision has been made, the examiner may not issue another certificate at a later date without completing an entirely new exam.

Testing: Height and Weight

At some point during the exam, the driver's height (in feet and inches) and weight (in pounds) need to be measured and recorded in the "Testing" section of the form.

The physical qualification standards do not include any maximum or minimum height and weight requirements. The examiner should consider height and weight factors as part of the overall driver medical fitness for duty.

NOTE: Trained assistants may measure height and weight. However, the examiner must take responsibility for all documented test results.

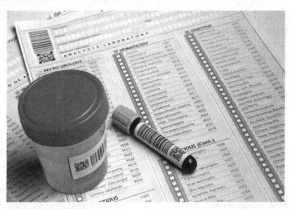

Testing: Urinalysis

The next portion of the exam form concerns the results of urinalysis and is to be completed by the medical examiner.

Urinalysis	Sp. Gr.	Protein	Blood	Sugar
Urinalysis is required. Numerical readings must be recorded.	1.02	7	Neg.	97

The examiner must perform a urinalysis (dip stick), testing for specific gravity, protein (proteinuria), blood (hematuria), and sugar (glycosuria).

NOTE: Trained assistants may obtain urine specimens and record test results. However, the examiner must sign the exam form, thereby taking responsibility for and attesting to the validity of all documented test results.

Abnormal urine readings may indicate a need for further testing. The examiner is expected to evaluate the test results and other physical findings to determine the next step. For example, sugar in the urine may prompt the examiner to obtain a blood glucose test. If the urinalysis, combined with other medical findings, indicates the potential for renal dysfunction, the examiner should obtain additional tests and/or consultation.

The examiner must document all additional test results and include the results in comments on the exam form, including whether or not the health of the driver affects his or her safe driving ability. Any additional medical reports that were obtained should be attached to the exam form.

Q: Must the examiner test for drug use?
A: No, testing for controlled substances is not a required part of the driver examination process (though it used to be). Drug testing is regulated under other parts of the driver safety regulations. However, if the medical examiner suspects a need for drug/alcohol testing, the examiner is advised to contact the FMCSA or the motor carrier for information on drug and alcohol testing under 49 CFR Part 382. Specific questions may be directed to an FMCSA field office or the FMCSA headquarters at (800) 832-5660.

Q: Can a DOT drug test also be performed on the urine sample?
A: Yes. When a DOT drug test is required at the same time as a DOT medical exam, a single urine specimen may be used for both. However, the urine to be used for the DOT test must be sealed into the specimen bottles before any remaining

THE EXAM

65

urine is taken or used for the physical exam (e.g., for glucose testing). See §40.13.

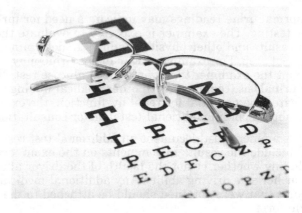

Testing: Vision

The vision portion of the exam report form is to be completed by the medical examiner.

Vision

Standard is at least 20/40 acuity (Snellen) in each eye with or without correction. At least 70° field of vision in horizontal meridian measured in each eye. The use of corrective lenses should be noted on the Medical Examiner's Certificate.

Acuity	Uncorrected	Corrected	Horizontal Field of Vision
Right Eye:	20/<u>20</u>	20/____	Right Eye: <u>120</u> degrees
Left Eye:	20/<u>20</u>	20/____	Left Eye: <u>120</u> degrees
Both Eyes:	20/<u>20</u>	20/____	

	Yes	No
Applicant can recognize and distinguish among traffic control signals and devices showing red, green, and amber colors	⊗	○
Monocular vision	○	⊗
Referred to ophthalmologist or optometrist?	○	⊗
Received documentation from ophthalmologist or optometrist?	○	⊗

When completing the vision section of the form, the examiner should:

- Use standard Snellen values, such as "20/20";

- Have drivers who wear corrective lenses for driving wear corrective lenses for testing;

- Evaluate drivers who wear contact lenses for good tolerance and adaptation to contact lens usage;

- Assess the ability to recognize and distinguish among red, yellow, and green traffic signals (true color perception deficiencies are rarely disqualifying); and

- If needed, request a vision exam by an ophthalmologist or optometrist (the form includes areas to record the referral and to indicate if results were received). Note that a specialist vision exam may be required for obtaining and renewing a medical exemption, or may be necessary when specialized diagnostic equipment is needed.

NOTE: Trained assistants may perform vision screening tests and record the results. However, the medical examiner must sign the exam form, thereby taking responsibility for and attesting to the validity of all documented test results.

Disqualifying visual conditions:
- **Monocular vision,**
- **Use of contact lenses when one lens corrects distant vision and the other corrects near vision,**
- **Use of telescopic lenses, or**
- **Failing to meet any part of the vision testing criteria with one eye or both eyes.**
Drivers with monocular vision may qualify for up to one year under the alternate vision standard in §391.44.

THE EXAM

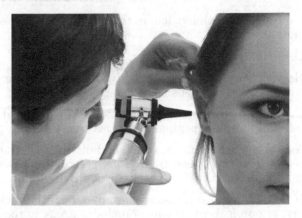

Testing: Hearing

The hearing portion of the exam form is to be completed by the medical examiner.

Hearing
Standard: Must first perceive whispered voice at not less than 5 feet OR average hearing loss of less than or equal to 40 dB, in better ear (with or without hearing aid).

Check if hearing aid used for test: ☐ Right Ear ☐ Left Ear ☒ Neither

Whisper Test Results   Right Ear   Left Ear

Record distance *(in feet)* from driver at which a forced
whispered voice can first be heard   4   4

OR

Audiometric Test Results

Right Ear			Left Ear		
500 Hz	1000 Hz	2000 Hz	500 Hz	1000 Hz	2000 Hz
30	33	35	40	43	50

Average (right):	32.6	Average (left):	44.3

To satisfy the federal hearing standard, the driver must successfully complete one hearing test with one ear. Both tests may not be necessary. The driver must:

- First perceive a forced, whispered voice **in one ear** at not less than five feet, OR

- Not have an average hearing loss **in one ear** greater than 40 decibels (dB) at 500 hertz (Hz), 1,000 Hz, and 2,000 Hz.

If the driver:	then the other test:
passed the initial hearing test	should NOT be administered, because the driver's hearing meets the standard.
failed the initial hearing test	should be administered.

Hearing Aids

A driver may use a hearing aid to meet the standard. However, the driver will usually have to go to an audiologist or hearing-aid center for testing with appropriate equipment because the audiometer used in most non-ear-specialty practices is not designed to test a person who is wearing a hearing aid.

The examiner must check the appropriate box(es) to indicate if a hearing aid was used for testing.

➢ **A driver who must use a hearing aid to qualify is required to use a hearing aid while driving, and should carry a spare power source.**

Entering Hearing Test Results

Numerical hearing-test results are to be recorded as follows:

a) For the **forced-whisper test**: The distance, in feet, at which a whispered voice is first heard, with separate values for the right and left ears.

THE EXAM

b) For the **audiometric test**: The hearing loss in dB for 500 Hz, 1,000 Hz, and 2,000 Hz, as well as the average, according to the American National Standards Institute (ANSI) standard Z24.5-1951.

NOTE: International Organization for Standardization (ISO) audiometric test results can be converted to ANSI results by:

• Subtracting 14 dB from ISO for 500 Hz.

• Subtracting 10 dB from ISO for 1,000 Hz.

• Subtracting 8.5 dB from ISO for 2,000 Hz.

NOTE: Trained assistants may perform hearing tests and record the results. However, the medical examiner must sign the form, thereby taking responsibility for and attesting to the validity of all documented test results.

Hearing Test Example

Hearing
Standard: Must first perceive whispered voice at not less than 5 feet OR average hearing loss of less than or equal to 40 dB, in better ear (with or without hearing aid).

Check if hearing aid used for test: ☐ Right Ear ☐ Left Ear ☒ Neither

Whisper Test Results   Right Ear   Left Ear

Record distance *(in feet)* from driver at which a forced
whispered voice can first be heard   4   4

OR

Audiometric Test Results

Right Ear			Left Ear		
500 Hz	1000 Hz	2000 Hz	500 Hz	1000 Hz	2000 Hz
30	33	35	40	43	50

Average (right):	32.6	Average (left):	44.3

In the image above, the examiner has documented the test results for both hearing tests and indicated that a hearing aid was not used. The forced-whisper test was

70

administered first, and the driver could not hear the forced whisper until he/she was four feet away. This did not meet the minimum five-foot standard in both ears. Therefore, the medical examiner also administered an audiometric test, resulting in:

- Right ear = 30 + 33 + 35 = 98/3 = 32.6 = PASS

- Left ear = 40 + 43 + 50 = 133/3 = 44.3 = FAIL

The hearing standard was met because the average hearing loss in the right ear was less than 40 dB when measured with an audiometer.

This driver passed one hearing test in one ear, thus meeting the qualification standard for hearing.

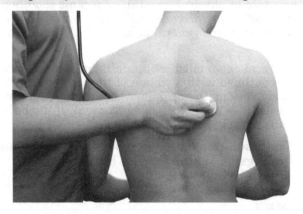

Physical Examination

The next section of the exam form concerns the actual physical examination of the driver and is to be completed by the medical examiner.

IV. The Medical Exam

PHYSICAL EXAMINATION

The presence of a certain condition may not necessarily disqualify a driver, particularly if the condition is controlled adequately, is not likely to worsen, or is readily amenable to treatment. Even if a condition does not disqualify a driver, the Medical Examiner may consider deferring the driver temporarily. Also, the driver should be advised to take the necessary steps to correct the condition as soon as possible, particularly if neglecting the condition could result in a more serious illness that might affect driving.

Check the body systems for abnormalities.

Body System	Normal	Abnormal	Body System	Normal	Abnormal
1. General	○	⊗	8. Abdomen	⊗	○
2. Skin	⊗	○	9. Genito-urinary system including hernias	⊗	○
3. Eyes	⊗	○	10. Back/Spine	⊗	○
4. Ears	⊗	○	11. Extremities/joints	⊗	○
5. Mouth/throat	⊗	○	12. Neurological system including reflexes	⊗	○
6. Cardiovascular	⊗	○	13. Gait	⊗	○
7. Lungs/chest	⊗	○	14. Vascular system	⊗	○

Discuss any abnormal answers in detail in the space below and indicate whether it would affect the driver's ability to operate a CMV. Enter applicable item number before each comment.

Markedly overweight; rest of exam unremarkable. Does not interfere with ability to drive. Recommended seeing PCP for diet and weight management.

(Attach additional sheets if necessary)

The general purpose of the physical exam is to detect the presence of physical, mental, or organic conditions that may affect the driver's ability to operate a CMV safely. Safety of the general public is the primary consideration.

The physical exam must, at a minimum, cover the body systems outlined in this section of the exam form. For each body system, the examiner is to mark "Abnormal" if abnormalities are detected, or "Normal" if the body system is normal.

➢ **The examiner must document any abnormal findings on the form even if they are not disqualifying.**

Comments

Any comments entered below the list of 14 body systems should begin with the number of the body system to which it applies, such as "3" for eyes or "14" for vascular system. The comments should:

• Indicate whether or not the abnormality affects driving ability;

• Indicate if additional evaluation is needed;

- Include a copy of any supplementary medical evaluation that was obtained;

- Document the examiner's discussion with the driver, which may include advice to seek additional evaluation of a condition that is not disqualifying but could, if neglected, worsen and affect driving ability; and

- Indicate whether or not the body has compensated for an organic disease adequately to meet physical qualification requirements.

Overview of Physical Exam

The following is an overview of how the examiner is to complete the physical exam.

1. General Appearance

The examiner is to observe and note on the form:

- Any abnormalities with posture, limps, or tremors;

- Driver emotions and overall appearance; and

- Driver demeanor and whether responses to questions indicate a potential impact on safe driving.

The examiner should observe:

- Whether the driver is markedly overweight. If yes, what are the clinical and safety implications when integrated with all other findings?

- Whether there are signs of current alcohol or drug abuse. If yes, the driver should be referred to a specialist for evaluation. After successful counseling and/or treatment, a driver may be considered for certification as long as no lasting limitations exist that could interfere with the ability to safely operate a CMV.

2. Skin

If an abnormality is observed, the examiner must determine whether the condition or treatment requires long-term follow-up and monitoring to ensure that the

THE EXAM

73

disease is stabilized, and whether the treatment is effective and well tolerated.

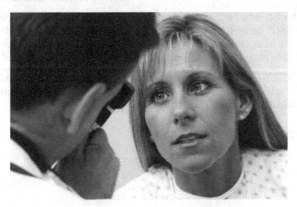

3. Eyes

At a minimum, the examiner should check for pupillary equality, reaction to light and accommodation, eye movement, eye muscle imbalance, extraocular movement, nystagmus, and exophthalmos.

If an abnormality is found, the examiner will determine if the abnormality interferes with driving ability or indicates that additional evaluation, perhaps by a specialist, is needed to assess the nature and severity of the underlying condition.

NOTE: Special diagnostic equipment may be needed to assess a driver with a known diagnosis or who is at risk for retinopathy, cataracts, aphakia, glaucoma, or macular degeneration. Referral to a vision specialist may be required.

4. Ears

The examiner should check for evidence of any aural disease or condition. At a minimum, this includes checking for:

• Scarring of the tympanic membrane,

- Obstruction of the external canal, and

- Perforated eardrums.

The examiner will need to decide if any abnormalities might account for hearing loss or a disturbance in balance, and whether the driver should consult with a primary care provider or hearing specialist for possible treatment that might improve hearing test results.

> **The presence of some hearing disorders, such as Meniere's disease, may interfere significantly with driving ability and the performance of other CMV driver tasks. In this case, guidelines recommend not to certify the driver.**

5. Mouth and Throat

If an abnormality is observed, the examiner must determine whether the condition or treatment requires long-term follow-up and monitoring to ensure that the disease is stabilized, and whether the treatment is effective and well tolerated.

6. Cardiovascular

The examiner should:

- Check the heart for murmurs, extra sounds, enlargement, and a pacemaker or implantable cardioverter defibrillator; and

- Check the lower extremities for pitting edema and other signs of cardiac disease.

The examiner will need to investigate any signs of cardiovascular disease and decide on proper treatment and monitoring.

? Q: Can the examiner order work restrictions for a driver with heart trouble?
A: No, work restrictions are not allowed. The driver must be able to perform all job-related tasks, including lifting, to be certified.

THE EXAM

7. Lungs / Chest

The examiner must check for:

- Abnormal chest-wall expansion, respiratory rate, and breath sounds including wheezes or the sound of fluid in the lungs;

- Impaired respiratory function and bluish skin due to a lack of oxygen in the blood;

- Clubbing of the fingers and other signs of pulmonary disease in the extremities; and

- A respiratory problem that in any way could interfere with safe CMV operation.

The driver may need to have additional pulmonary function tests and/or have a specialist evaluation to adequately assess respiratory function.

8. Abdomen

The examiner must check for:

- Enlarged liver and spleen, masses, bruits, and significant weakness of the abdominal wall muscles;

- Tenderness and unusual bowel sounds; and

- Any other abnormal findings that might suggest a condition that could interfere with safe CMV operation.

A certification decision should not be made until the cause is confirmed and treatment has been shown to be adequate, effective, and safe.

9. Genito-Urinary System

The examiner must check for hernias and evaluate any hernia that causes the driver discomfort, to determine the extent to which it might interfere with safe driving. Further testing and evaluation may be required.

If the urinalysis is abnormal, further testing may be needed to rule out underlying medical problems.

NOTE: A driver who has not provided a urine specimen cannot be certified.

10. Back/Spine

The examiner must check the musculoskeletal system for previous surgery, deformities, limitations of motion, and tenderness. The examiner should determine whether the driver has a diagnosis or signs of a condition known to be associated with acute episodes of transient muscle weakness, poor muscular coordination, abnormal sensations, decreased muscular tone, and/or pain.

11. Extremities/Joints

The examiner must check for:

- Loss, impairment, or deformity of an arm, hand, finger, leg, foot, or toe;

- A perceptible limp;

- Enough grasp in the upper limbs to maintain steering-wheel grip;

- Enough mobility and strength in the lower limbs to operate pedals properly;

- Signs of progressive musculoskeletal conditions, such as atrophy, weakness, or low muscle tone; and

- Clubbing or excess fluid that may indicate the presence of an underlying heart, lung, or vascular condition.

NOTE: If a driver is found to be medically qualified except for the loss or impairment of a limb, the driver may be qualified subject to obtaining an SPE certificate. The SPE program is intended only for individuals with "fixed deficits" of the extremities, not progressive diseases.

THE EXAM

77

IV. The Medical Exam

12. Neurological System

The examiner must check for:

- Impaired equilibrium, coordination, and speech patterns;
- Lack of muscle control (ataxia);
- Deep tendon reflexes that are asymmetrical;
- Patellar reflexes;
- Babinski's reflex;
- Sensory or positional abnormalities; and
- Any abnormal findings suggesting a condition that might interfere with safe CMV operation.

If problems are found, a certification decision should not be made until the cause is confirmed and treatment has been shown to be adequate, effective, and safe.

13. Gait

If an abnormality is observed, the examiner must determine whether the condition or treatment requires long-term follow-up and monitoring to ensure that the condition or disease is stabilized, and whether the treatment is effective and well tolerated.

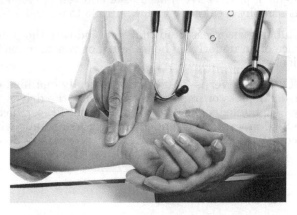

14. Vascular (Blood) System

The examiner must check for:

- Abnormal pulse and amplitude,

- Carotid or arterial bruits (abnormal sounds caused by obstructions),

- Varicose veins, and

- Pulse in the foot.

A diagnosis of arterial disease should lead to an evaluation for other cardiovascular diseases. This may require additional testing and/or an exam from a specialist.

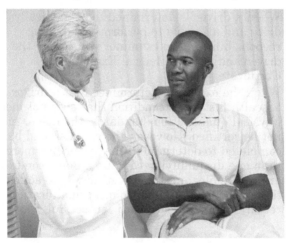

THE EXAM

Determining Certification Status

The FMCSA relies on the medical examiner to assess and determine if a CMV driver meets the physical qualification requirements in §391.41. In some cases, the examiner will also consider any reports and recommendations from the primary care provider and/or specialists treating the driver to supplement his or her examination and ensure adequate medical assessment.

IV. The Medical Exam

The medical examiner is responsible for making the certification decision and signing the Medical Examination Report form. A Medical Examiner's Certificate is issued to drivers who are determined to be medically fit for duty.

The examiner's certification decision is limited to the certification and disqualification options printed on the Medical Examination Report form.

> The *maximum* time for which a driver can be certified is two years. Drivers may be certified for less than that, however.

Certification Status

✔ When a driver is determined to be medically fit to drive and also able to perform non-driving responsibilities, the examiner will certify the driver and issue a Medical Examiner's Certificate.

✘ When the examiner determines that a driver has a health history or condition that does not meet physical qualification standards, the driver must not be certified. However, the exam should be completed to determine if the driver has more than one disqualifying condition. Some conditions are reversible, and the driver may take actions that will enable him/her to meet qualification requirements if treatment is successful.

The examiner must discuss the certification decision with the driver to ensure that the driver understands that decision:

Certification Decision	Topics to be Included in the Discussion

Certified	• The reason for any periodic monitoring and/or a shortened examination interval.
	
	• Additional requirements associated with certification.
	
	• The certificate expiration:
	  − That it occurs at midnight on the expiration date, and
	  − That there is no grace period.

Disqualified	• The reason for disqualification.
	
	• The steps that can be taken to meet certification standards.
	
	• For temporary disqualification:
	  − The reason (condition or medication),
	  − The length of waiting period,
	  − The conditions that could restart the waiting period, and
	  − The list of any documentation the driver is to provide to the examiner.

THE EXAM

Certification Options

The medical examiner decides:

• Whether a driver meets the physical qualification requirements (whether federal or state), and

• How often a driver has to repeat the physical exam to stay certified.

The only other constraints or requirements that the examiner can place on the driver are those in the "Medical Examiner Determination" section of the Medical Examination Report form and at the top of the Medical Examiner's Certificate. An examiner may not, for example, try to limit the amount of weight that drivers may lift by adding some type of restriction to the certificate.

IV. The Medical Exam

The certification period cannot be more than two years, but it can be less. The FMCSA has certain "recommended best practices" for the length of certification, but the examiner is not required to certify a driver for any longer than he/she deems necessary to adequately monitor a driver's medical fitness.

State or federal?

The examiner must complete either page 4 *or* page 5 of the exam form:

- **Page 4 (federal) is the default for most commercial drivers who are examined in accordance with the Federal Motor Carrier Safety Regulations (Secs. 391.41-391.49).**

- **Page 5 (state) is only to be used for drivers who are not fully qualified for interstate operations but who may qualify to drive in-state only (intrastate) by virtue of a state-issued variance or exemption. For example, a state may have a "grandfather" provision or a special diabetes exemption program for its in-state drivers.**

Pages 4 and 5 of the Medical Examination Report form correspond to the first two options on the Medical Examiner's Certificate. If the examiner completes page 5 and restricts the driver to in-state operations, for example, then the examiner should check the second option on the Certificate, indicating that the driver is certified "with any applicable State variances."

Meets Standards

When a driver is fully certified under the Federal Motor Carrier Safety Regulations, the examiner must:

- Complete page 4 of the exam form;

- Mark the box labeled "Meets standards in 49 CFR 391.41; qualifies for 2 year certificate"; and

- Verify that the expiration date on the certificate is two years from the date of the exam.

MEDICAL EXAMINER DETERMINATION (Federal)

Use this section for examinations performed in accordance with the Federal Motor Carrier Safety Regulations (49 CFR 391.41-391.49):

○ Does not meet standards *(specify reason)*: _____

⊗ Meets standards in 49 CFR 391.41; qualifies for 2-year certificate

○ Meets standards, but periodic monitoring required *(specify reason)*: _____

Needs Periodic Monitoring

If a driver is qualified but needs monitoring more often than every two years, the examiner must:

- Mark the box labeled "Meets standards, but periodic monitoring required *(specify reason)*: _____";

- Note the reason for periodic monitoring;

- Indicate the length of certification by checking 3 months, 6 months, or 1 year, or by checking "Other" and writing in the time frame (e.g., 18 months); and

- Calculate the expiration date from the date of the exam.

> ⊗ Meets standards, but periodic monitoring required *(specify reason)*:   Stage 2 hypertension
> Driver qualified for: ⊗ 3 months   ○ 6 months   ○ 1 year   ○ other *(specify)*: _____

Required to Wear Corrective Lenses And/Or Hearing Aid

If a driver needs corrective lenses and/or a hearing aid to meet the vision and/or hearing standards, then the examiner must specify – as a requirement for certification – that the driver must wear corrective lenses and/or a hearing aid while driving a CMV.

The examiner must mark the "Wearing corrective lenses" and/or "Wearing hearing aid" option on the form.

A driver can be certified for up to two years even if required to wear corrective lenses and/or a hearing aid.

> ⊗ Meets standards in 49 CFR 391.41; qualifies for 2-year certificate
> ○ Meets standards, but periodic monitoring required *(specify reason)*: _____
> Driver qualified for: ○ 3 months   ○ 6 months   ○ 1 year   ○ other *(specify)*: _____
> ☒ Wearing corrective lenses   ☒ Wearing hearing aid   ☐ Accompanied by a waiver/exemption *(specify type)*:

THE EXAM

83

IV. The Medical Exam

Needs SPE Certificate

If a driver needs a Skill Performance Evaluation (SPE) Certificate due to a limb impairment, the examiner must mark the SPE box. By marking the SPE option, the examiner is certifying that the driver:

- Fails to meet one or more of the limb requirements of §391.41(b)(1) or (2);

- Meets all other physical requirements cited in §391.41(b); and

- Must have both a valid SPE certificate and Medical Examiner's Certificate to drive.

The medical examiner starts the SPE program application process by first determining if the driver is otherwise medically qualified. A copy of the Medical Examination Report form is required with initial and renewal SPE applications. An SPE certificate is issued for 2 years.

⊗ Meets standards in 49 CFR 391.41 qualifies for 2-year certificate	
◯ Meets standards, but periodic monitoring required *(specify reason)*: _____	
Driver qualified for: ◯ 3 months ◯ 6 months ◯ 1 year ◯ other *(specify)*: _____	
☐ Wearing corrective lenses ☐ Wearing hearing aid ☐ Accompanied by a waiver/exemption *(specify type)*: _____	
☒ Accompanied by a Skill Performance Evaluation (SPE) Certificate ☐ Qualified by operation of 49 CFR 391.64 *(Federal)*	

Needs a Federal Exemption

Drivers may apply for an exemption from one or more federal medical standards. An exemption, if granted, allows someone to drive a commercial vehicle in interstate commerce despite a disqualifying medical condition. The FMCSA is currently issuing exemptions from its standards for hearing and epilepsy. The maximum certification period is generally one year, to allow for monitoring. Drivers using the Federal Vision Exemption program or the Grandfather provision in §391.64 must be qualified under the alternation vision standard under §391.44 no later than March 21, 2023.

The medical examiner starts the exemption program application process by first determining if the driver is otherwise medically qualified except for the condition for which an exemption will be applied (e.g., monocular vision, epilepsy, etc.). A copy of the Medical Examination Report form is required with both the initial and renewal federal exemption applications.

⊗ Meets standards, but periodic monitoring required *(specify reason)*:	Monocular vision	
Driver qualified for: ○ 3 months ○ 6 months ⊗ 1 year ○ other *(specify)*:		
□ Wearing corrective lenses □ Wearing hearing aid ☒ Accompanied by a waiver/exemption *(specify type)*:	Vision exemption	

By marking "Accompanied by a waiver/exemption" and writing in the federal exemption type, the examiner is certifying that the driver:

• Fails to meet the standards for vision (§391.41(b)(10)), hearing (§391.41(b)(11)), or epilepsy/seizures (§391.41(b)(8));

• Meets all other physical requirements cited in §391.41(b); and

• Must also have a valid federal medical exemption certificate to drive.

Grandfathered Under Vision/Diabetes Waiver Study Program (§391.64)

Section 391.64 offered an exemption from the vision and diabetes standards for a small number of drivers who have been continuously participating in an FMCSA waiver study program since March 31, 1996. (NOTE: The diabetes waiver study program is terminated effective Nov. 19, 2019. The Federal vision exemption program and grandfathered drivers must be qualified under the alternate vision standard in 391.44 no later than March 21, 2023.) By checking the box labeled "Qualified by operation of 49 CFR 391.64," the examiner certified that the driver:

• Presented documentation of participation in one of the studies;

IV. The Medical Exam

- Continues to meet the requirements of §391.64; and

- Is otherwise medically fit for duty.

⊗ Meets standards, but periodic monitoring required *(specify reason)*: Vision waiver study program	

Driver qualified for: ◯ 3 months   ◯ 6 months   ⊗ 1 year   ◯ other *(specify)*: _____
☐ Wearing corrective lenses   ☐ Wearing hearing aid   ☐ Accompanied by a waiver/exemption *(specify type)*: _____
☐ Accompanied by a Skill Performance Evaluation (SPE) Certificate   ☒ Qualified by operation of *49 CFR 391.64 (Federal)*

Qualifies for Intra-City Zone Exemption (§391.62)

Section 391.62 offers an exemption from most medical standards for drivers who:

- Have suffered from an otherwise disqualifying medical condition since about 1988, and that condition has not substantially worsened;

- Have been driving within an exempt intra-city zone since November 18, 1987; and

- Do not transport hazardous materials requiring placarding.

Exempt intra-city zones are geographical areas defined in the regulations. See the definition in §390.5.

> According to §391.43(d), "any driver authorized to operate a commercial motor vehicle within an exempt intra city zone ... shall furnish the examining medical examiner with a copy of the medical findings that led to the issuance of the first certificate of medical examination which allowed the driver to operate a commercial motor vehicle wholly within an exempt intra city zone."

By checking the "Driving within an exempt intra-city zone" option, the examiner is certifying that:

- The driver is otherwise medically fit for duty except for the exempted condition;

- The exempted condition remains stable; and

- The driver remains in medical compliance with the requirements of §391.62.

☐ Accompanied by a Skill Performance Evaluation (SPE) Certificate   ☐ Qualified by operation of <u>49 CFR 391.64</u> *(Federal)*

☒ Driving within an exempt intracity zone *(see <u>49 CFR 391.62</u>) (Federal)*

☐ Determination pending *(specify reason):* _____

Determination Pending

The exam form includes an option for the examiner to designate the exam results as "pending" if more information is needed to make a qualification decision. The examiner must specify the date when the driver must return to the medical exam office for follow-up. The qualification decision can be delayed for as many as 45 days. If the decision is not completed by then, the exam must be re-done. Specifically, if the decision is not updated on the National Registry website on or before the 45-day expiration date, the FMCSA will notify the examiner and the driver in writing that the examination is no longer valid and that the driver will have to be re-examined.

While an exam is "pending," the driver's existing medical certificate (if any) will remain valid until its expiration date.

☒ Determination pending *(specify reason):*   Awaiting results of polysomnogram

    ☒ Return to medical exam office for follow-up on *(must be 45 days or less):*   07/01/2016

➣   **When an exam result is placed into "determination pending" status, a medical examiner's certificate should NOT be issued. The driver must rely on his or her existing certificate until the certification decision can be made. If the driver's existing certificate expires before then, the driver is no longer qualified to drive.**

A Medical Examination Report Form may only be amended while in "determination pending" status for situations where new information (such as a test result) has been received or there has been a change in the driver's medical status since the initial exam. The reason for the amendment must be entered on the form.

Meets standards, but periodic monitoring required *(specify reason)*: Monitor for sleep apnea

Driver qualified for: ○ 3 months ○ 6 months ⊗ 1 year ○ other *(specify)*: _____

☐ Wearing corrective lenses ☐ Wearing hearing aid ☐ Accompanied by a waiver/exemption *(specify type)*: _____
☐ Accompanied by a Skill Performance Evaluation (SPE) Certificate ☐ Qualified by operation of 49 CFR 391.64 *(Federal)*
☐ Driving within an exempt intracity zone *(see 49 CFR 391.62) (Federal)*

☒ Determination pending *(specify reason)*: Awaiting results of polysomnogram

  ☒ Return to medical exam office for follow-up on *(must be 45 days or less)*: 07/01/2016

  ☒ Medical Examination Report amended *(specify reason)*: Negative results received; issued 1-year cert

  (if amended) Medical Examiner's Signature: *Jamie Wilson* Date: 07/01/2016

☐ Incomplete examination *(specify reason)*: _____

Incomplete Exam

When a physical examination is not completed for any reason (e.g., a driver decides he/she does not want to continue with the exam and leaves), other than situations resulting in "determination pending," the examiner must check the "Incomplete exam" box and specify the reason.

☒ Incomplete examination *(specify reason)*: Driver walked out of exam when questioned about marijuana use

State Variances

When a driver is unable to be fully qualified for interstate operations but may qualify to drive in-state only (intrastate) by virtue of a state-issued variance or exemption, the examiner may complete page 5 of the exam form – instead of page 4 – to document a state-level determination. For example, a state may have a "grandfather" provision or a special exemption program for its in-state drivers. Some states do not offer any in-state exemptions or variances, so page 5 would not be used in those states. It's up to the medical examiner to be familiar with the variances and exemptions that are offered in the state and to use page 5 appropriately.

MEDICAL EXAMINER DETERMINATION (State)

Use this section for examinations performed in accordance with the Federal Motor Carrier Safety Regulations (49 CFR 391.41-391.49) with any applicable State variances (which will only be valid for intrastate operations):

○ Does not meet standards in 49 CFR 391.41 with any applicable State variances *(specify reason)*: _____

○ Meets standards in 49 CFR 391.41 with any applicable State variances

⊗ Meets standards, but periodic monitoring required *(specify reason)*: Diabetes

Driver qualified for: ○ 3 months ○ 6 months ⊗ 1 year ○ other *(specify)*: _____
☐ Wearing corrective lenses ☐ Wearing hearing aid ☒ Accompanied by a waiver/exemption *(specify type)*: DPS Diabetes Exemption

The top half of the "Medical Examiner Determination (State)" section is used to document the driver's certification status:

- **Does not meet standards in 49 CFR 391.41 with any applicable State variances:** This option is selected when a driver is not qualified to operate in-state. The examiner must provide an explanation of why the driver doesn't meet the standards.

- **Meets standards in 49 CFR 391.41 with any applicable State variances:** This option is selected when a driver is deemed qualified and will be issued a 2-year certificate.

- **Meets standards, but periodic monitoring is required:** This option is used when a driver is found to be qualified but needs monitoring more frequently than every 2 years. The examiner must provide an explanation of why periodic monitoring is required and must select the corresponding timeframe.

- **Corrective lenses/hearing aid/waivers/ exemptions:** The examiner must select any checkboxes that apply to the driver's certification, e.g., must wear corrective lenses, grandfathered, must carry a state-issued waiver, etc.

Note that page 5 of the exam form does *not* have an option for placing an exam into a "pending" status. Drivers must either be certified or disqualified at the time of the exam.

Disqualification

Any driver who does not meet one or more of the physical qualification standards in §391.41 must be disqualified except as noted above. When a driver is disqualified, the examiner should:

- Complete the physical exam of the driver,

- Discuss the reason(s) for disqualification, and

- Discuss any steps that can be taken to meet the certification standards.

IV. The Medical Exam

The medical examiner must disqualify any driver who:

- Fails to meet a physical qualification requirement cited in the standards (e.g., vision, hearing, epilepsy, or insulin use); or

- Has a medical condition that endangers the health and safety of the driver and the public.

The examiner must document the decision to disqualify someone on the Medical Examination Report form by:

- Marking the "Does not meet standards" box;

- Noting the reason for disqualification; and

- Documenting the discussion with the driver explaining the rationale for the disqualification decision.

A medical examiner's certificate must NOT be issued if the driver was disqualified.

➤ **Before a disqualified driver can return to CMV driving, a medical examiner must find the driver to be medically fit for duty.**

Completing the Exam Form

The final step in completing the exam form is for the examiner to sign the form and add identifying information, as well as the certificate expiration date (if a certificate is issued).

I have performed this evaluation for certification. I have personally reviewed all available records and recorded information pertaining to this evaluation, and attest that to the best of my knowledge, I believe it to be true and correct.	

Medical Examiner's Signature: _Jamie Wilson_

Medical Examiner's Name *(please print or type)*: Jamie L. Wilson, PA

Medical Examiner's Address: 189 N. State   City: Salt Lake City   State: UT   Zip Code: 84001

Medical Examiner's Telephone Number: (801) 555-5555   Date Certificate Signed: 5/23/2016

Medical Examiner's State License, Certificate, or Registration Number: ME56789   Issuing State: UT

☐ MD ☐ DO ☒ Physician Assistant ☐ Chiropractor ☐ Advanced Practice Nurse
☐ Other Practitioner *(specify)*: _____

National Registry Number: 0123456789 | Medical Examiner's Certificate Expiration Date: 5/23/2018

Note the following on this portion of the exam form:

- **Date Certificate Signed:** This may or may not be the same as the exam date. For example, if a completed exam was placed into "pending" status (for up to 45 days), the certificate would not be signed until the certification decision is actually made.

- **National Registry Number:** This is the identification number for the medical examiner as listed in the National Registry of Certified Medical Examiners.

- **Medical Examiner's Certificate Expiration Date:** This is the date the driver's new medical certificate will expire, not the expiration date of the examiner's state certificate or license. This date should be calculated based on the date the driver's certificate was signed, not necessarily the date of the exam.

Issuance of Medical Examiner's Certificate

The medical examiner is required to issue a Medical Examiner's Certificate to any driver who is medically qualified to operate a CMV in accordance with §391.41(b). The certificate must be documented on form MCSA-5876, as shown in §391.43 (see also Chapter 5).

The examiner:

- *Must* give the original certificate to the driver; and

- *Must* give a copy to a prospective or current employer who requests one.

THE EXAM

IV. The Medical Exam

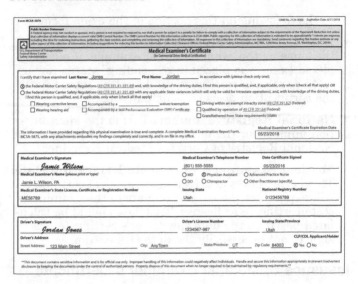

When completing the certificate, the examiner is expected to:

1. Ensure that the name of the driver matches the name on the Medical Examination Report form.

2. Mark the proper type of certification based on the type of exam that was completed, either:

   - Fully based on federal standards for interstate travel, corresponding to page 4 of the exam form; or

   - Based on federal standards but with any applicable state variances, valid for intrastate travel only and corresponding to page 5 of the exam form.

3. Mark any certification requirement that applies (any selection made here should correspond with the same selection on page 4 or 5 of the exam form):

    ❏ Wearing corrective lenses

    ❏ Wearing hearing aid

    ❏ Accompanied by a _____ waiver or exemption (the examiner must specify the type of waiver or exemption required, e.g., vision, hearing, etc.)

    ❏ Accompanied by a Skill Performance Evaluation (SPE) Certificate

    ❏ Driving within an exempt intracity zone (49 CFR 391.62)

    ❏ Qualified by operation of 49 CFR 391.64

    ❏ Grandfathered from state requirements

4. Enter the Medical Examiner's Certificate Expiration Date, which is the date the driver's certificate will expire (not the expiration date of the medical examiner's occupational license). Note that the date of the medical exam does not appear on the certificate. Verify that the expiration date does not exceed the certification interval (maximum certification period is two years).

5. Sign and date the certificate and complete the medical examiner information. This includes the number and state of the examiner's occupational license/certificate/registration, as well as the examiner's identification number in the National Registry of Certified Medical Examiners. The examiner may choose to enter the driver's information as well (other than the signature), or may have the driver complete those sections (see step 6 below).

> **The "National Registry Number" is required for any DOT exams conducted on interstate CMV drivers.**

THE EXAM

6. Have the driver sign the certificate and enter his/ her address and licensing information, and compare this with other information provided by the driver. The driver (or medical examiner) must indicate:

   - **CLP/CDL Applicant/Holder:** Whether the driver holds a commercial driver's license (CDL) or commercial learner's permit (CLP) or intends to apply for one.

   - **Driver's License Number:** The driver's license number, whether a CDL/CLP or not.

   - **Issuing State/Province:** The name or abbreviation of the issuing state or Canadian province of the driver's license.

When a driver is stopped for a roadside inspection, the inspector may verify the contents of the certificate by contacting the examiner at the telephone number shown on the certificate.

V. Forms & Recordkeeping

Medical Examination Report

While performing a DOT medical examination, the examiner is required to complete a Medical Examination Report form, commonly referred to as the "long" form. Detailed instructions for how the exam form is to be completed are discussed in Chapter 4.

Federal regulations (§391.43) state that "the medical examination shall be performed, and its results shall be recorded on the Medical Examination Report Form, MCSA–5875," as illustrated on the following pages.

Form MCSA-5875

OMB No.: 2126-0006   Expiration Date: 03/31/2025

Public Burden Statement
A Federal agency may not conduct or sponsor, and a person is not required to respond to, nor shall a person be subject to a penalty for failure to comply with a collection of information subject to the requirements of the Paperwork Reduction Act unless that collection of information displays a currently valid OMB Control Number. The OMB Control Number for this information collection is 2126-0006. Public reporting for this collection of information is estimated to be approximately 25 minutes per response, including the time for reviewing instructions, gathering the data needed, and completing and reviewing the collection of information. All responses to this collection of information are mandatory. Send comments regarding this burden estimate or any other aspect of this collection of information, including suggestions for reducing this burden to: Information Collection Clearance Officer, Federal Motor Carrier Safety Administration, MC-RRA, 1200 New Jersey Avenue, SE, Washington, D.C. 20590.

U.S. Department of Transportation
Federal Motor Carrier
Safety Administration

Medical Examination Report Form
(for Commercial Driver Medical Certification)

MEDICAL RECORD #
_____
(or sticker)

SECTION 1. Driver Information *(to be filled out by the driver)*

PERSONAL INFORMATION

Last Name: _____   First Name: _____   Middle Initial: ____   Date of Birth: _____   Age: ____

Street Address: _____   City: _____   State/Province: _____   Zip Code: _____

Driver's License Number: _____   Issuing State/Province: _____   Phone: _____

E-Mail *(optional)*: _____   CLP/CDL Applicant/Holder*: ○ Yes ○ No

Driver ID Verified By**: _____

Has your USDOT/FMCSA medical certificate ever been denied or issued for less than 2 years?   ○ Yes ○ No ○ Not Sure

*CLP/CDL Applicant/Holder: See instructions for definitions.   **Driver ID Verified By: Record what type of photo ID was used to verify the identity of the driver, e.g., CDL, driver's license, passport.

DRIVER HEALTH HISTORY

Have you ever had surgery? If "yes," please list and explain below.   ○ Yes ○ No ○ Not Sure

Are you currently taking medications *(prescription, over-the-counter, herbal remedies, diet supplements)*?   ○ Yes ○ No ○ Not Sure
If "yes," please describe below.

(Attach additional sheets if necessary)

This document contains sensitive information and is for official use only. Improper handling of this information could negatively affect individuals. Handle and secure this information appropriately to prevent inadvertent disclosure by keeping the documents under the control of authorized persons. Properly dispose of this document when no longer required to be maintained by regulatory requirements.

Rev 3/29/2022

Page 1

Form MCSA-5875   OMB No.: 2126-0006   Expiration Date: 03/31/2025

Last Name: _____ First Name: _____ DOB: _____ Exam Date: _____

DRIVER HEALTH HISTORY (continued)

Do you have or have you ever had:	Yes	No	Not Sure		Yes	No	Not Sure
1. Head/brain injuries or illnesses *(e.g., concussion)*	○	○	○	16. Dizziness, headaches, numbness, tingling, or memory loss	○	○	○
2. Seizures/epilepsy	○	○	○	17. Unexplained weight loss	○	○	○
3. Eye problems *(except glasses or contacts)*	○	○	○	18. Stroke, mini-stroke (TIA), paralysis, or weakness	○	○	○
4. Ear and/or hearing problems	○	○	○	19. Missing or limited use of arm, hand, finger, leg, foot, toe	○	○	○
5. Heart disease, heart attack, bypass, or other heart problems	○	○	○	20. Neck or back problems	○	○	○
6. Pacemaker, stents, implantable devices, or other heart procedures	○	○	○	21. Bone, muscle, joint, or nerve problems	○	○	○
7. High blood pressure	○	○	○	22. Blood clots or bleeding problems	○	○	○
8. High cholesterol	○	○	○	23. Cancer	○	○	○
9. Chronic (long-term) cough, shortness of breath, or other breathing problems	○	○	○	24. Chronic (long-term) infection or other chronic diseases	○	○	○
10. Lung disease *(e.g., asthma)*	○	○	○	25. Sleep disorders, pauses in breathing while asleep, daytime sleepiness, loud snoring	○	○	○
11. Kidney problems, kidney stones, or pain/problems with urination	○	○	○	26. Have you ever had a sleep test *(e.g., sleep apnea)*?	○	○	○
12. Stomach, liver, or digestive problems	○	○	○	27. Have you ever spent a night in the hospital?	○	○	○
13. Diabetes or blood sugar problems	○	○	○	28. Have you ever had a broken bone?	○	○	○
Insulin used	○	○	○	29. Have you ever used or do you now use tobacco?	○	○	○
14. Anxiety, depression, nervousness, other mental health problems	○	○	○	30. Do you currently drink alcohol?	○	○	○
15. Fainting or passing out	○	○	○	31. Have you used an illegal substance within the past two years?	○	○	○
				32. Have you ever failed a drug test or been dependent on an illegal substance?	○	○	○

Other health condition(s) not described above: ○ Yes ○ No ○ Not Sure

Did you answer "yes" to any of questions 1-32? If so, please comment further on those health conditions below: ○ Yes ○ No ○ Not Sure

(Attach additional sheets if necessary)

CMV DRIVER'S SIGNATURE

I certify that the above information is accurate and complete. I understand that inaccurate, false or missing information may invalidate the examination and my Medical Examiner's Certificate, that submission of fraudulent or intentionally false information is a violation of 49 CFR 390.35, and that submission of fraudulent or intentionally false information may subject me to civil or criminal penalties under 49 CFR 390.37 and 49 CFR 386 Appendices A and B.

Driver's Signature: _____   Date: _____

SECTION 2. Examination Report *(to be filled out by the medical examiner)*

DRIVER HEALTH HISTORY REVIEW

Review and discuss pertinent driver answers and any available medical records. Comment on the driver's responses to the "health history" questions that may affect the driver's safe operation of a commercial motor vehicle (CMV).

(Attach additional sheets if necessary)

Page 2

Form MCSA-5875 OMB No.: 2126-0006 Expiration Date: 03/31/2025

Last Name:	First Name:	DOB:	Exam Date:

TESTING

Pulse Rate: _____ Pulse rhythm regular: ○ Yes ○ No

Height: ___ feet ___ inches Weight: ___ pounds

Blood Pressure	Systolic	Diastolic
Sitting		
Second reading (optional)		

Urinalysis	Sp. Gr.	Protein	Blood	Sugar
Urinalysis is required. Numerical readings must be recorded.				

Other testing if indicated

Protein, blood, or sugar in the urine may be an indication for further testing to rule out any underlying medical problem.

Vision
Standard is at least 20/40 acuity (Snellen) in each eye with or without correction. At least 70° field of vision in horizontal meridian measured in each eye. The use of corrective lenses should be noted on the Medical Examiner's Certificate.

Acuity	Uncorrected	Corrected	Horizontal Field of Vision
Right Eye:	20/____	20/____	Right Eye: ____ degrees
Left Eye:	20/____	20/____	Left Eye: ____ degrees
Both Eyes:	20/____	20/____	

	Yes	No
Applicant can recognize and distinguish among traffic control signals and devices showing red, green, and amber colors	○	○
Monocular vision	○	○
Referred to ophthalmologist or optometrist?	○	○
Received documentation from ophthalmologist or optometrist?	○	○

Hearing
Standard: Must first perceive whispered voice at not less than 5 feet OR average hearing loss of less than or equal to 40 dB, in better ear (with or without hearing aid).

Check if hearing aid used for test: ☐ Right Ear ☐ Left Ear ☐ Neither

Whisper Test Results   Right Ear Left Ear
Record distance (in feet) from driver at which a forced
whispered voice can first be heard   _____ _____

OR

Audiometric Test Results
Right Ear: Left Ear:

500 Hz	1000 Hz	2000 Hz	500 Hz	1000 Hz	2000 Hz
____	____	____	____	____	____

Average (right): _____   Average (left): _____

PHYSICAL EXAMINATION

The presence of a certain condition may not necessarily disqualify a driver, particularly if the condition is controlled adequately, is not likely to worsen, or is readily amenable to treatment. Even if a condition does not disqualify a driver, the Medical Examiner may consider deferring the driver temporarily. Also, the driver should be advised to take the necessary steps to correct the condition as soon as possible, particularly if neglecting the condition could result in a more serious illness that might affect driving.

Check the body systems for abnormalities.

Body System	Normal	Abnormal	Body System	Normal	Abnormal
1. General	○	○	8. Abdomen	○	○
2. Skin	○	○	9. Genito-urinary system including hernias	○	○
3. Eyes	○	○	10. Back/spine	○	○
4. Ears	○	○	11. Extremities/joints	○	○
5. Mouth/throat	○	○	12. Neurological system including reflexes	○	○
6. Cardiovascular	○	○	13. Gait	○	○
7. Lungs/chest	○	○	14. Vascular system	○	○

Discuss any abnormal answers in detail in the space below and indicate whether it would affect the driver's ability to operate a CMV. Enter applicable item number before each comment.

(Attach additional sheets if necessary)

Page 3

Form MCSA-5875   OMB No.: 2126-0006   Expiration Date: 03/31/2025

Last Name: _____   First Name: _____   DOB: _____   Exam Date: _____

Please complete only one of the following (Federal or State) Medical Examiner Determination sections:

MEDICAL EXAMINER DETERMINATION (Federal)

Use this section for examinations performed in accordance with the Federal Motor Carrier Safety Regulations (49 CFR 391.41-391.49):

○ Does not meet standards *(specify reason):* _____

○ Meets standards in 49 CFR 391.41; qualifies for 2-year certificate

○ Meets standards, but periodic monitoring required *(specify reason):* _____

　　Driver qualified for: ○ 3 months   ○ 6 months   ○ 1 year   ○ other *(specify):* _____

　　☐ Wearing corrective lenses　　☐ Wearing hearing aid　　☐ Accompanied by a waiver/exemption *(specify type):* _____

　　☐ Accompanied by a Skill Performance Evaluation (SPE) Certificate　　☐ Qualified by operation of 49 CFR 391.64 *(Federal)*

　　☐ Driving within an exempt intracity zone *(see 49 CFR 391.62) (Federal)*

○ Determination pending *(specify reason):* _____

　　☐ Return to medical exam office for follow-up on *(must be 45 days or less):* _____

　　☐ Medical Examination Report amended *(specify reason):* _____

　　　　(if amended) Medical Examiner's Signature: _____   Date: _____

○ Incomplete examination *(specify reason):* _____

> **If the driver meets the standards outlined in 49 CFR 391.41, then complete a Medical Examiner's Certificate as stated in 49 CFR 391.43(h), as appropriate.**

I have performed this evaluation for certification. I have personally reviewed all available records and recorded information pertaining to this evaluation, and attest that, to the best of my knowledge, I believe it to be true and correct.

Medical Examiner's Signature: _____

Medical Examiner's Name *(please print or type):* _____

Medical Examiner's Address: _____   City: _____   State: _____   Zip Code: _____

Medical Examiner's Telephone Number: _____   Date Certificate Signed: _____

Medical Examiner's State License, Certificate, or Registration Number: _____   Issuing State: _____

☐ MD　☐ DO　☐ Physician Assistant　☐ Chiropractor　☐ Advanced Practice Nurse

☐ Other Practitioner *(specify):* _____

National Registry Number: _____   Medical Examiner's Certificate Expiration Date: [_____]

Page 4

V. Forms & Recordkeeping

Form MCSA-5875

OMB No.: 2126-0006   Expiration Date: 03/31/2025

Last Name:	First Name:	DOB:	Exam Date:

MEDICAL EXAMINER DETERMINATION (State)

Use this section for examinations performed in accordance with the Federal Motor Carrier Safety Regulations (49 CFR 391.41-391.49) with any applicable State variances (which will only be valid for intrastate operations):

○ Does not meet standards in 49 CFR 391.41 with any applicable State variances *(specify reason):*

○ Meets standards in 49 CFR 391.41 with any applicable State variances

○ Meets standards, but periodic monitoring required *(specify reason):*

Driver qualified for: ○ 3 months ○ 6 months ○ 1 year ○ other *(specify):*

☐ Wearing corrective lenses ☐ Wearing hearing aid ☐ Accompanied by a waiver/exemption *(specify type):*

☐ Accompanied by a Skill Performance Evaluation (SPE) Certificate ☐ Grandfathered from State requirements *(State)*

> **If the driver meets the standards outlined in 49 CFR 391.41, with applicable State variances, then complete a Medical Examiner's Certificate, as appropriate.**

I have performed this evaluation for certification. I have personally reviewed all available records and recorded information pertaining to this evaluation, and attest that, to the best of my knowledge, I believe it to be true and correct.

Medical Examiner's Signature:

Medical Examiner's Name *(please print or type):*

Medical Examiner's Address:	City:	State:	Zip Code:

Medical Examiner's Telephone Number: Date Certificate Signed:

Medical Examiner's State License, Certificate, or Registration Number: Issuing State:

☐ MD ☐ DO ☐ Physician Assistant ☐ Chiropractor ☐ Advanced Practice Nurse

☐ Other Practitioner *(specify):*

National Registry Number:	Medical Examiner's Certificate Expiration Date:

Page 5

Instructions MCSA-5875

Instructions for Completing the Medical Examination Report Form (MCSA-5875)

I. Step-By-Step Instructions

Driver:

Section 1: Driver Information

- **Personal Information:** Please complete this section using your name as written on your driver's license, your current address and phone number, your date of birth, age, driver's license number and issuing state.

  ◦ **CLP/CDL Applicant/Holder:** Check "yes" if you are a commercial learner's permit (**CLP**) or commercial driver's license (**CDL**) holder, or are applying for a CLP or CDL. CDL means a license issued by a State or the District of Columbia which authorizes the individual to operate a class of a commercial motor vehicle (**CMV**). A CMV that requires a CDL is one that: (1) has a gross combination weight rating or gross combination weight of 26,001 pounds or more inclusive of a towed unit with a gross vehicle weight rating (**GVWR**) or gross vehicle weight (**GVW**) of more than 10,000 pounds; or (2) has a GVWR or GVW of 26,001 pounds or more; or (3) is designed to transport 16 or more passengers, including the driver; or (4) is used to transport either hazardous materials requiring hazardous materials placards on the vehicle or any quantity of a select agent or toxin.

  ◦ **Driver ID Verified By:** The Medical Examiner/staff completes this item and notes the type of photo ID used to verify the driver's identity such as, commercial driver's license, driver's license, or passport, etc.

  ◦ **Has your USDOT/FMCSA medical certificate ever been denied or issued for less than two years?** Please check the correct box "yes" or "no" and if you aren't sure check the "not sure" box.

- **Driver Health History:**

  ◦ **Have you ever had surgery:** Please check "yes" if you have ever had surgery and provide a written explanation of the details (type of surgery, date of surgery, etc.)

  ◦ **Are you currently taking medications (prescription, over-the-counter, herbal remedies, diet supplements):** Please check "yes" if you are taking any diet supplements, herbal remedies, or prescription or over the counter medications. In the box below the question, indicate the name of the medication and the dosage.

  ◦ **#1-32:** Please complete this section by checking the "yes" box to indicate that you have, or have ever had, the health condition listed or the "No" box if you have not. Check the "not sure" box if you are unsure.

  ◦ **Other Health Conditions not described above:** If you have, or have had, any other health conditions not listed in the section above, check "Yes" and in the box provided and list those condition(s).

  ◦ **Any yes answers to questions #1-32 above:** If you have answered "yes" to any of the questions in the Driver Health History section above, please explain your answers further in the box below the question. For example, if you answered "yes" to question #5 regarding heart disease, heart attack, bypass, or other heart problem, indicate which type of heart condition. If you checked "yes" to question #23 regarding cancer, indicate the type of cancer. Please add any information that will be helpful to the Medical Examiner.

- **CMV Driver Signature and Date:** Please read the certification statement, sign and date it, indicating that the information you provided in Section 1 is accurate and complete.

FORMS/RECORDS

Medical Examiner:

Section 2: Examination Report

- **Driver Health History Review:** Review answers provided by the driver in the driver health history section and discuss any "yes" and "not sure" responses. In addition, be sure to compare the medication list to the health history responses ensuring that the medication list matches the medical conditions noted. Explore with the driver any answers that seem unclear. Record any information that the driver omitted. As the Medical Examiner conducting the driver's physical examination you are required to complete the entire medical examination even if you detect a medical condition that you consider disqualifying, such as deafness. Medical Examiners are expected to determine the driver's physical qualification for operating a commercial vehicle safely. Thus, if you find a disqualifying condition for which a driver may receive a Federal Motor Carrier Safety Administration medical exemption, please record that on the driver's Medical Examiner's Certificate, Form MCSA-5876, as well as on the Medical Examination Report Form, MCSA-5875.

- **Testing:**

  ○ **Pulse rate and rhythm, height, and weight:** record these as indicated on the form.

  ○ **Blood Pressure:** record the blood pressure (systolic and diastolic) of the driver being examined. A second reading is optional and should be recorded if found to be necessary.

  ○ **Urinalysis:** record the numerical readings for the specific gravity, protein, blood and sugar.

  ○ **Vision:** The current vision standard is provided on the form. When other than the Snellen chart is used, give test results in Snellen-comparable values. When recording distance vision, use 20 feet as normal. Record the vision acuity results and indicate if the driver can recognize and distinguish among traffic control signals and devices showing red, green, and amber colors; has monocular vision; has been referred to an ophthalmologist or optometrist; and if documentation has been received from an ophthalmologist or optometrist.

  ○ **Hearing:** The current hearing standard is provided on the form. Hearing can be tested using either a whisper test or audiometric test. Record the test results in the corresponding section for the test used.

- **Physical Examination:** Check the body systems for abnormalities and indicate normal or abnormal for each body system listed. Discuss any abnormal answers in detail in the space provided and indicate whether it would affect the driver's ability to safely operate a commercial motor vehicle.

In this next section, you will be completing either the Federal or State determination, not both.

- **Medical Examiner Determination (Federal):** Use this section for examinations performed in accordance with the FMCSRs (49 CFR 391.41-391.49). Complete the medical examiner determination section completely. When determining a driver's physical qualification, please note that English language proficiency (49 CFR part 391.11: General qualifications of drivers) is not factored into that determination.

  ○ **Does not meet standards:** Select this option when a driver is determined to be not qualified and provide an explanation of why the driver does not meet the standards in 49 CFR 391.41.

  ○ **Meets standards in 49 CFR 391.41; qualifies for 2-year certification:** Select this option when a driver is determined to be qualified and will be issued a 2-year Medical Examiner's Certificate.

- ° **Meets standards, but periodic monitoring is required:** Select this option when a driver is determined to be qualified but needs periodic monitoring and provide an explanation of why periodic monitoring is required. Select the corresponding time frame that the driver is qualified for, and if selecting "other" specify the time frame.

  — **Determination that driver meets standards:** Select all categories that apply to the driver's certification (e.g., wearing corrective lenses, accompanied by a waiver/exemption, driving within an exempt intracity zone, etc.).

- ° **Determination pending:** Select this option when more information is needed to make a qualification decision and specify a date, on or before the 45 day expiration date, for the driver to return to the medical exam office for follow-up. This will allow for a delay of the qualification decision for as many as 45 days. If the disposition of the pending examination is not updated via the National Registry on or before the 45 day expiration date, FMCSA will notify the examining medical examiner and the driver in writing that the examination is no longer valid and that the driver is required to be re-examined.

  — **MER amended:** A Medical Examination Report Form (MER), MCSA-5875, may only be amended while in determination pending status for situations where new information (e.g., test results, etc.) has been received or there has been a change in the driver's medical status since the initial examination, but prior to a final qualification determination. Select this option when a Medical Examination Report Form, MCSA-5875, is being amended; provide the reason for the amendment, sign and date. In addition, initial and date any changes made on the Medical Examination Report Form, MCSA-5875. A Medical Examination Report Form, MCSA-5875, cannot be amended after an examination has been in determination pending status for more than 45 days or after a final qualification determination has been made. The driver is required to obtain a new physical examination and a new Medical Examination Report Form, MCSA-5875, should be completed.

- ° **Incomplete examination:** Select this when the physical examination is not completed for any reason (e.g., driver decides they do not want to continue with the examination and leaves) other than situations outlined under determination pending.

- ° **Medical Examiner information, signature and date:** Provide your name, address, phone number, occupation, license, certificate, or registration number and issuing state, national registry number, signature and date.

- ° **Medical Examiner's Certificate Expiration Date:** Enter the date the **driver's** Medical Examiner's Certificate (MEC) expires.

- **Medical Examiner Determination (State):** Use this section for examinations performed in accordance with the FMCSRs (49 CFR 391.41-391.49) with any applicable State variances (which will only be valid for intrastate operations). Complete the medical examiner determination section completely.

  - ° **Does not meet standards in** 49 CFR 391.41 **with any applicable State variances:** Select this option when a driver is determined to be not qualified and provide an explanation of why the driver does not meet the standards in 49 CFR 391.41 with any applicable State variances.

  - ° **Meets standards in** 49 CFR 391.41 **with any applicable State variances:** Select this option when a driver is determined to be qualified and will be issued a 2-year Medical Examiner's Certificate.

FORMS/RECORDS

V. Forms & Recordkeeping

Instructions MCSA-5875

- ○ **Meets standards, but periodic monitoring is required:** Select this option when a driver is determined to be qualified but needs periodic monitoring and provide an explanation of why periodic monitoring is required. Select the corresponding time frame that the driver is qualified for, and if selecting "other" specify the time frame.

  — **Determination that driver meets standards:** Select all categories that apply to the driver's certification (e.g., wearing corrective lenses, accompanied by a waiver/exemption, etc.).

- ○ **Medical Examiner information, signature and date:** Provide your name, address, phone number, occupation, license, certificate, or registration number and issuing state, national registry number, signature and date.

- ○ **Medical Examiner's Certificate Expiration Date:** Enter the date the **driver's** Medical Examiner's Certificate (MEC) expires.

II. **If updating an existing exam, you must resubmit the new exam results, via the Medical Examination Results Form, MCSA-5850, to the National Registry, and the most recent dated exam will take precedence.**

III. **To obtain additional information regarding this form go to the Medical Program's page on the Federal Motor Carrier Safety Administration's website at** http://www.fmcsa.dot.gov/regulations/medical.

Recordkeeping: The Exam Form

• The examiner is to retain the Medical Examination Report form and related medical records for a minimum of 3 years.

• The examiner may need to provide a copy of the form to any driver who is applying for, or renewing, a Skill Performance Evaluation (SPE) certificate or other medical waiver or exemption.

• For information on a motor carrier's use and retention of the exam form, see "Use of the Medical Examination Report form" below.

Medical Examiner's Certificate

The medical examiner must issue a completed Medical Examiner's Certificate – also known as a "med" card, "wallet" card, or "fed med" card – to any driver who is considered to be medically qualified to drive a CMV. The certificate "shall be completed in accordance with the following Form MCSA-5876," as shown here:

Form MCSA-5876   OMB No.: 2126-0006   Expiration Date: 03/31/2025

Public Burden Statement

A Federal agency may not conduct or sponsor, and a person is not required to respond to, nor shall a person be subject to a penalty for failure to comply with a collection of information subject to the requirements of the Paperwork Reduction Act unless that collection of information displays a current valid OMB Control Number. The OMB Control Number for this information collection is 2126-0006. Public reporting for this collection of information is estimated to be approximately one minute per response, including the time for reviewing instructions, gathering the data needed, and completing and reviewing the collection of information. All responses to this collection of information are mandatory. Send comments regarding this burden estimate or any other aspect of this collection of information, including suggestions for reducing this burden to: Information Collection Clearance Officer, Federal Motor Carrier Safety Administration, MC-RRA, 1200 New Jersey Avenue, SE, Washington, D.C. 20590.

U.S. Department of Transportation
Federal Motor Carrier
Safety Administration

Medical Examiner's Certificate
(for Commercial Driver Medical Certification)

I certify that I have examined **Last Name:** _____ **First Name:** _____ In accordance with *(please check only one):*

- ○ the Federal Motor Carrier Safety Regulations (49 CFR 391.41-391.49) and, with knowledge of the driving duties, I find this person is qualified, and, if applicable, only when *(check all that apply)* **OR**
- ○ the Federal Motor Carrier Safety Regulations (49 CFR 391.41-391.49) with any applicable State variances (which will only be valid for intrastate operations), and, with knowledge of the driving duties, I find this person is qualified, and, if applicable, only when *(check all that apply):*

☐ Wearing corrective lenses	☐ Accompanied by a _____ waiver/exemption	☐ Driving within an exempt intracity zone (49 CFR 391.62) (Federal)
☐ Wearing hearing aid	☐ Accompanied by a Skill Performance Evaluation (SPE) Certificate	☐ Qualified by operation of 49 CFR 391.64 (Federal)
		☐ Grandfathered from State requirements (State)

The information I have provided regarding this physical examination is true and complete. A complete Medical Examination Report Form, MCSA-5875, with any attachments, embodies my findings completely and correctly, and is on file in my office.

Medical Examiner's Signature _____

Medical Examiner's Telephone Number _____

Date Certificate Signed _____

Medical Examiner's Certificate Expiration Date _____

Medical Examiner's Name *(please print or type)* _____

○ MD   ○ Physician Assistant   ○ Advanced Practice Nurse
○ DO   ○ Chiropractor   ○ Other Practitioner *(specify)*

Medical Examiner's State License, Certificate, or Registration Number _____

Issuing State _____ **National Registry Number** _____

Driver's Signature _____

Driver's License Number _____

Issuing State/Province _____

Driver's Address

Street Address: _____ City: _____ State/Province: _____ Zip Code: _____

CLP/CDL Applicant/Holder
○ Yes   ○ No

This document contains sensitive information and is for official use only. Improper handling of this information could negatively affect individuals. Handle and secure this information appropriately to prevent inadvertent disclosure by keeping the documents under the control of authorized persons. Properly dispose of this document when no longer required to be maintained by regulatory requirements.

Rev 3/29/22

Recordkeeping: The Certificate

- The examiner must provide the original Medical Examiner's Certificate to any driver who was examined and found medically fit for duty.

- The examiner must retain a copy of the certificate for at least 3 years.

- The examiner must provide a copy to a prospective or current employer upon request.

- In most cases, the driver must carry the certificate while operating a CMV.* The certificate may be:

  - The original certificate,

  - A copy of the original certificate, or

  - A reduced-size (but legible) copy of the original certificate (e.g., wallet size).

- The certificate may be laminated, if desired.

*NOTE: Interstate commercial driver's license (CDL) and commercial learner's permit (CLP) holders are exempt from needing to carry the medical certificate for more than 15 days after it was issued (see below for details).

Certificate recordkeeping on and after June 23, 2025
Beginning June 23, 2025, medical examiners must only issue a medical certificate to non-CDL/CLP drivers. For each CDL/CLP driver examined, medical certification information will be sent directly to the FMCSA and then to the state licensing agency shortly after the exam, and the motor carrier must obtain and use a driving record as proof of medical certification, instead of a medical certificate.

FORMS/RECORDS

Driver Recordkeeping

A driver's proper use and retention of the medical certificate or waiver/exemption documentation depends on whether the driver:

- Is involved in interstate (across state lines) commerce or intrastate (in-state-only) commerce;

- Holds a commercial driver's license (CDL) or commercial learner's permit (CLP); and/or

- Has received a medical variance (i.e., waiver or exemption).

Interstate CDL/CLP Drivers Subject to Federal Medical Standards

These drivers must provide each new medical certificate to their state driver licensing agency, before the previous certificate expires. This should be done within five days of receiving the certificate, if possible.

These drivers must carry the certificate (or a copy) for up to 15 days after it was issued, or until the state licensing agency updates the driving record (MVR) with information from the certificate. The states have 10 days to update the MVR after receiving the certificate. Once the MVR is updated, the driver no longer has to carry the certificate.

On and after June 23, 2025, these drivers will no longer receive medical certificates unless requested.

Interstate Non-CDL/CLP Drivers Subject to Federal Medical Standards

These drivers must carry a valid medical certificate at all times while driving a commercial motor vehicle.

Interstate CDL/CLP Drivers Granted a Medical Variance

These drivers must provide each new medical certificate to their state driver licensing agency, before the previous certificate expires. This should be done within five days of receiving the certificate, if possible. The FMCSA will notify the state directly of the medical variance.

These drivers must:

• Carry the certificate (or a copy) for up to 15 days after it was issued, or until the state licensing agency updates the driving record (MVR) with information from the certificate. The states have 10 days to update the MVR after receiving the certificate. Once the MVR is updated, the driver no longer has to carry the certificate.

• Carry the original (or a copy) of the medical variance documentation at all times when on duty. This is in addition to the CDL itself, which should carry a "V" (variance) restriction code.

On and after June 23, 2025, these drivers will no longer receive medical certificates unless requested.

Interstate Non-CDL/CLP Drivers Granted a Medical Variance

These drivers must carry a valid medical certificate – in addition to documentation of the variance – at all times while driving a commercial motor vehicle.

Intrastate Drivers

Intrastate drivers are subject to state medical standards, including standards for medical exams and documentation of those exams. In many cases, the requirements will be the same as for interstate drivers, as described above. In some cases, the state may have additional exemptions or may require use of state-specific forms. Check with your state for details.

FORMS/RECORDS

109

Employer Recordkeeping

For Interstate CDL/CLP Drivers Subject to Federal Medical Standards

Verify and document that the driver's medical examiner was listed on the National Registry of Certified Medical Examiners at the time of the exam. Retain this documentation for at least three years. The "document" may simply be a note verifying that the carrier checked the Registry.

Once a driver has submitted his or her medical certificate to the state licensing agency, then:

- Obtain a copy of the driver's driving record (MVR) from that state within 15 days of the date the certificate was issued (the state has 10 days to process the medical card and update the driver's record). Until that point, keep a copy of the medical certificate on file to prove that the driver is currently certified. It is recommended that the certificate be retained for three years.

- Verify that the MVR contains current medical certification information and that the driver's status is "certified." If the state fails in its obligation to provide medical certification information on the MVR, it is recommended that you keep the medical certificate on file beyond the initial 15-day period, as proof of certification until an updated MVR can be obtained.

- Keep the MVR on file for at least three years. Note, however, that the initial MVR(s) obtained at the time of hire must be kept until three years after employment ends.

- Obtain a new MVR whenever the medical certificate is updated, or as needed to perform a DOT-required annual review.

- Do not use an interstate CDL/CLP driver whose MVR does not contain information about his/her medical certification status, except within the 15-day grace period mentioned above (unless the state has failed to provide the required medical information on its MVRs).

- Do not use an interstate CDL/CLP driver whose MVR indicates that he/she is "not certified."

NOTE: Beginning June 23, 2025, the MVR will be the *only* official proof that a CDL/CLP driver is medically certified. These drivers will not be issued medical certificates on and after that date, and motor carriers will need to obtain a new MVR within days after each medical exam. Also beginning June 23, 2025, motor carriers will no longer need to verify that the medical examiners for these drivers are listed on the National Registry.

For Interstate Non-CDL/CLP Drivers Subject to Federal Medical Standards

Keep on file the original or copy of the driver's medical certificate. Each new certificate can be removed from the file after three years.

Verify and document that the driver's medical examiner was listed on the National Registry of Certified Medical Examiners at the time of the exam. Retain this documentation for at least three years. The "document" may simply be a note verifying that the carrier checked the Registry.

For Interstate CDL/CLP Drivers Granted a Medical Variance

Follow the above procedures for drivers who do not hold a medical variance, but also keep on file the original or copy of the variance documentation. Such documentation must be kept for at least three years from its creation date.

FORMS/RECORDS

111

For Interstate Non-CDL/CLP Drivers Granted a Medical Variance

Keep on file the original or copy of the driver's medical certificate and documentation of the medical variance. These documents must be kept for at least three years from their creation date.

Verify and document that the driver's medical examiner was listed on the National Registry of Certified Medical Examiners at the time of the exam. Retain this documentation for at least three years. The "document" may simply be a note verifying that the carrier checked the Registry.

For Intrastate Drivers Subject to State Medical Standards

Comply with the state's documentation requirements. In many cases, the requirements will be the same as for interstate drivers, as described above.

Use of the Medical Examination Report Form

The Medical Examination Report form, also known as the "long" form, is used by the medical examiner to document the DOT medical exam.

The examiner may supply this form, or the motor carrier can supply the form to help ensure that it is the most current form available. Use of an incorrect form could lead to a medically unqualified driver being certified because the criteria and instructions on the form may be outdated.

The long form – unlike the driving record and/or medical exam certificate (wallet card) – is not a required element of a driver file. According to federal regulations, the medical examiner is required to keep the original exam form on file at his/her office for three years. The regulations do not prohibit motor carriers from obtaining the form. If a motor carrier or driver obtains a copy, they are not required to retain it in the driver's file.

As a best practice, many carriers request copies of the DOT exam forms to review, to help ensure that their drivers are medically qualified. However, federal law (HIPAA) says that healthcare providers cannot release medical forms or discuss a driver's condition without the patient's written consent, so a driver could legally refuse to allow his or her employer to see the exam form. The same privacy laws would not apply to a motor carrier that obtains the form directly from a driver.

Another federal law – the *Americans with Disabilities Act* (ADA) – requires that employee or applicant medical information be kept confidential (see 29 CFR §1630). Under the ADA, medical information like the DOT medical long form cannot be stored in a personnel file or any file resembling a personnel file (including a driver qualification file). The exam form must be kept in a separate, confidential medical file away from any personnel-type file. This does not apply to the medical certificate, which must be kept in the driver's qualification file.

> Be aware that some states may require drivers to provide a copy of the medical exam report form to the state. This falls under state laws and is not prohibited by federal laws or regulations.

Privacy, ADA, and HIPAA

Just because DOT medical exams are required for most commercial motor vehicle drivers does not mean that federal privacy and non-discrimination laws do not apply. Such laws include:

* The *Americans with Disabilities Act* (ADA),

* The *Health Insurance Portability and Accountability Act* (HIPAA), and

* The *Genetic Information Nondiscrimination Act* (GINA).

FORMS/RECORDS

113

Among other things, these laws protect the confidentiality of drivers' medical exams and prevent motor carriers from discriminating against drivers with certain medical conditions.

Generally, HIPAA applies only to medical information from a healthcare provider or health plan, but not to medical information requested or obtained in the course of employment. Those medical exams or inquiries, such as evaluating a driver's fitness for duty, fall under the ADA. Finally, under GINA, employers cannot discriminate against an employee based on genetic information. Those protections are similar to laws prohibiting discrimination based on race, gender, national origin, and similar protected classes.

Obtaining the "Long" Exam Form

As noted previously, the long Medical Examination Report form that the medical examiner completes during the exam does NOT have to be obtained by the motor carrier. An FMCSA auditor will (or should) not expect to see the long form in a driver's files. Rather, FMCSA regulations say that the form is to be kept on file at the examiner's office.

Many motor carriers feel a need to review the "long form," however, to help ensure that the examiner did his or her job in qualifying the driver. FMCSA regulations do not prohibit motor carriers from obtaining the form, nor do they prohibit examiners from releasing the form, but other federal laws do affect how that form may be released.

HIPAA privacy rules apply to confidential medical information released by healthcare providers, among others. In general, medical examiners are not allowed to disclose a driver's protected health information without appropriate authorization from that individual.

Therefore, there are basically two ways in which a motor carrier can legally obtain the long examination form:

1. The carrier can have the driver authorize the medical facility to release the form to the carrier. The driver would have to sign a HIPAA-compliant release form (usually provided by the medical facility) and give that release to the healthcare provider, who could then release the medical exam form to the carrier.

2. The carrier can ask the driver to obtain the form from the examiner and provide it directly to the carrier. In this case, a release form would not be required.

Q: Can a carrier "force" a driver to provide his or her completed medical exam form as a condition of employment?
A: After a conditional offer of employment is made, a company may ask questions and make demands that are "job related and consistent with business necessity." It is recommended that motor carrier employers contact a human-resources professional or attorney to help ensure compliance with this ADA provision.

Q: Can an employer who spots an insurance claim through their company-sponsored health plan indicating that an employee had a certain medical condition use that information to order the employee to undergo a medical exam?
A: The short answer is "no" because any protected health information a HIPAA-covered employer gains through its group health plan must remain separate from the employer's typical employment duties. Such "firewalls" between the plan and the

FORMS/RECORDS

115

plan sponsor are necessary to prevent unauthorized use and disclosure of protected health information. The employer would also not be able to take any adverse employment action based on the health information that was obtained in this case, such as terminating or suspending the driver.

Once a motor carrier has the "long form," confidentiality and non-discrimination laws come into play.

Confidentiality

The ADA imposes very strict limitations on the use of medical information obtained from exams or other medical inquiries of applicants and employees. All such medical information must be collected and maintained on separate forms and in separate medical files, and must be treated as confidential medical records.

Though the medical certificate (which does not contain sensitive medical information) is usually a required part of a driver's qualification (DQ) file under DOT regulations, motor carriers must not place any medical-related material in an employee's *personnel* file. In particular, this includes the long Medical Examination Report form, which is generally full of confidential medical information.

> REMEMBER: The FMCSA does not require employers to have, review, or use the medical long form. Therefore, there are no DOT regulations protecting an employer who chooses to obtain and/or use the form.

Steps must be taken to guarantee the security of each employee's (including each driver's) medical information, including:

- Keeping the information in a separate medical file and in a separate, locked cabinet, apart from the location of the personnel files (or in a secure, password-protected electronic file); and

- Designating a specific person or persons to have access to the medical file.

Medical-related information must be kept confidential, but there are some narrow exceptions:

- Supervisors and managers may be informed about necessary restrictions on the work or duties of an employee and necessary accommodations.

- First aid and safety personnel may be informed, when appropriate, if the disability might need emergency treatment or if any specific procedures are needed in the case of fire or other evacuation.

- Government officials investigating compliance with the ADA and other federal and state laws prohibiting discrimination on the basis of disability should be provided relevant information on request. Other federal laws and regulations also may require disclosure of relevant medical information.

- Relevant information may be provided to state workers' compensation offices or "second injury" funds in accordance with state workers' compensation laws.

- Relevant information may be provided to insurance companies where the company requires a medical exam to provide health or life insurance for employees.

The ADA's confidentiality provisions include co-workers. Carriers should not explain to other employees that their co-worker is allowed to do something that generally is not permitted (such as have more breaks or work more in the warehouse) because he or she has a medical condition. Carriers may not disclose that an employee has a medical condition or is receiving a reasonable accommodation. Doing so amounts to a disclosure of the employee's medical condition. However, an employer certainly may respond to a question about why a co-worker is receiving what is perceived as "different" or "special" treatment by emphasizing that the company tries to assist any employee who experiences difficulties in the workplace.

FORMS/RECORDS

117

Rather than disclosing that an employee is receiving a reasonable accommodation, employers should focus on the importance of maintaining the privacy of all employees and emphasize that company policy is to refrain from discussing the work situation of any employee with co-workers.

Employers may also want to:

- Train employees on the requirements of equal employment opportunity laws, including the ADA; and/or

- Point out that many of the workplace issues encountered by employees are personal, and it is the company's policy to respect employee privacy.

An employer may allow an employee to voluntarily inform his or her co-workers of a medical condition and details related to the condition, but the employer is still limited in sharing this information with others and cannot coerce someone into disclosing medical information.

➢ **The basic rule is, employee medical information must be kept private!**

Discrimination

Claims of discrimination can easily arise when employers use medical information to make hiring and employment decisions. The ADA prohibits discrimination based on an actual or perceived disability.

Once a motor carrier obtains confidential medical information, it must be cautious in how it uses that information. Though motor carriers have an obligation to protect public safety, they cannot use medical or genetic information to discriminate against applicants with disabilities – or even genetic traits that may lead to disabilities in the future (that's where GINA comes in).

Some ways to help prevent claims of discrimination:

• Perform the DOT medical exam only after a conditional offer of employment has been extended to the driver. That way, medical information cannot be used to influence the employment decision.

• Do not screen out an individual with a disability – or a class of individuals with disabilities – unless the selection or screening criteria is shown to be job related and consistent with business necessity. Treat all drivers the same. Check with a human-resources professional or attorney to establish such criteria.

• Employers have a duty to provide reasonable accommodations for an individual with a disability. As one example, this might include pedal extenders for someone with a limb defect that prevents the ability to reach a vehicle's gas, clutch, and brake pedals. However, if an individual is unable to perform "essential job functions" and no accommodation can be made without causing undue hardship, the person may appropriately be deemed "not qualified" for the job. Again, check with a human-resources professional or attorney to determine if and when a reasonable accommodation is necessary.

FORMS/RECORDS

VI. Qualification Standards

The following are the FMCSA's medical qualification requirements, guidelines, and recommendations.

Vision

The standard: §391.41(b)(10)

A person is physically qualified to drive a commercial motor vehicle if that person has:

- Distant visual acuity of at least 20/40 in each eye without corrective lenses OR visual acuity separately corrected to 20/40 or better with corrective lenses;

- Distant binocular acuity of at least 20/40 in both eyes with or without corrective lenses;

- Field of vision of at least 70° in the horizontal meridian in each eye; and

- The ability to recognize the colors of traffic signals and devices showing standard red, green, and yellow.

Disqualifying visual conditions:
- **Monocular vision,**

- **Use of contact lenses when one lens corrects distant vision and the other corrects near vision,**

- **Use of telescopic lenses, or**

- **Failing to meet any part of the vision testing criteria with one eye or both eyes.**

Note: Drivers with monocular vision may qualify for up to 1 year based on vision in the better eye under the alternate vision standard by meeting the criteria and following the process in §391.44.

Key points:

- Vision is measured in each eye individually and both eyes together, using a standard "Snellen" eye chart.

- A medical examiner, ophthalmologist, or optometrist may perform and certify vision test results, but the medical examiner still must determine the driver's overall certification status.

- **If corrective lenses are used:** A driver who wears corrective lenses to pass the vision test must wear them while driving. The medical examiner has to mark the "wearing corrective lenses" checkbox on both the Medical Examination Report form and the medical examiner's certificate.

It is recommended that drivers who need to wear corrective lenses should carry a spare set of glasses. The driver avoids both stress and delay when lost or damaged eyeglasses or uncomfortable contact lenses can be replaced immediately.

Public safety considerations:

- Adequate central and peripheral vision are necessary for safe driving.

- The driver must perceive the relative distance of objects and react appropriately to vehicles in adjacent lanes or reflected in the mirrors, in order to pass, make lane changes, and avoid other vehicles on the road.

- The visual demands of driving are magnified by vehicles that have larger blind spots, longer turning radiuses, and increased stopping times.

Medications:

When prescribing medications for the eyes, the examiner needs to make sure the substance will have the desired effect without any visual and/or systemic side effects that interfere with safe driving (e.g., stinging, blurring, decreased night vision, sensitivity to glare, headache, or allergic reaction).

Agents used to treat:	include:
Age-related macular degeneration	• Antioxidants and zinc, and • Vascular endothelial growth factor (VEGF) inhibitors.
Allergic conjunctivitis	• Oral and topical antihistamines, • Topical decongestants, • Antihistamine/decongestant combinations, • Mast cell stabilizers, and • Topical non-steroidal anti-inflammatories.
Glaucoma	• Prostaglandin analogs, • Beta adrenergic blocking agents, • Carbonic anhydrase inhibitors, • Alpha agonists, • Cholinergic agonists, • Osmotic agents, and • Combinations.
Bacterial conjunctivitis	• Oral antibiotics, and • Topical antibiotics.
Dry eyes	• Lubricants, • Non-steroidal anti-inflammatories, and • Topical cyclosporine.

Physical exam:

During the eye exam, drivers should be asked about eye diseases or conditions such as retinopathy (retina damage), cataracts, aphakia (loss of a lens), glaucoma, and macular degeneration.

Medical examiners cannot diagnose these diseases or conditions because most do not have the equipment necessary to diagnose them. The following is a description of common eye diseases.

STANDARDS

Cataracts

Cataracts are a common cause of visual disturbances in the adult population. With cataracts, the lens of the eye slowly and progressively becomes opaque, distorting the optical passage of light to the retina resulting in diminished visual sharpness. Cataract formation can be accelerated by a number of conditions, including injury, diabetes, exposure to radiation, gout, and certain medications (steroids).

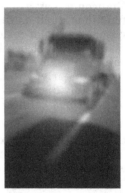

Glare, particularly during night driving in the face of oncoming headlights, may be an early symptom of cataracts. Glare, diminished overall sharpness, contrast, and color resolution are compounded by the light-scattering effect of the cataracts.

Treatment for cataracts is surgical removal and placement of the lens.

Glaucoma

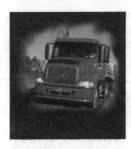

Glaucoma can harm peripheral vision. The abnormal regulation of pressure in the eye can result in gradual damage to optic nerve cells. The development of chronic elevated pressure is generally painless, and the gradual loss of peripheral visual field can progress significantly before symptoms are noticed.

Glaucoma may also affect a number of subtler visual functions, such as redirection of visual attention, night vision, and color vision. With glaucoma, eye-chart test results may not be affected, but peripheral field test results may show problems. Specialist examination may result in early detection and treatment before the onset of possibly disqualifying vision loss. Vision loss caused by glaucoma cannot be restored.

A therapeutic goal is to lower eye pressure to a level that preserves the existing neuronal cells and prevents further loss of peripheral vision. Strict use of prescribed eye medications is required for successful treatment; however, antiglaucoma agents may have side effects that impact vision and interfere with safe driving.

Macular Degeneration

Macular degeneration is a leading cause of untreatable legal blindness. Macular degeneration describes many eye diseases that impact the macula function and interfere with detailed, central vision. These diseases increase in prevalence with age, affecting some 30% of all Americans by age 70. For the majority of cases, macular degeneration is a slow process resulting in subtle visual defects; however, approximately 10% of cases are a "malignant" form of the disease and cause rapid loss of central vision.

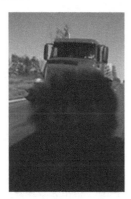

Peripheral vision is generally spared in macular degeneration. Therapeutic options are limited.

Macular degeneration causes noticeable signs and symptoms. Visual sharpness drops, recovery from bright lights takes longer, and eventually a partial or total loss of vision develops in the direction of attempted gaze. Snellen-type vision testing will detect diminishing central sharpness.

➤ **The use of telescopic lenses is not acceptable for commercial driving.**

Telescopic lenses redirect unaffected peripheral vision to compensate for lost central sharpness, resulting in a reduced peripheral field of vision.

STANDARDS

Retinopathy

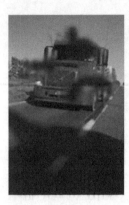

Non-inflammatory damage to the retina of the eye has many causes. The most common cause of retinopathy is diabetes, commonly developing after 5-7 years with diabetes. In many cases, the retinopathy does not progress beyond this stage; however, fluid leakage near the macula (diabetic macular edema) can create partial loss of central vision or cause hemorrhage in the eye which can obscure vision and eventually lead to retinal detachment and blindness.

Strict control of blood glucose, as well as medical control of related diseases (e.g., hypertension, renal disease, cardiac disease), may prevent or delay development of retinopathy.

Medical guidelines for the driver with diabetes include:

- Annual medical exams,
- Annual ophthalmologist or optometrist eye evaluation, and
- Disqualification if the driver is diagnosed with unstable proliferative retinopathy.

Other diseases can cause retinopathy, such as sickle-cell disease.

Required tests:

Required vision screening tests include central visual acuity, peripheral vision, and color vision.

Central visual acuity

The Snellen chart or the Titmus Vision Tester are used to measure central visual acuity. The standard is at least 20/40 in each eye and distant binocular visual acuity of at least 20/40.

➤ **Eyeglasses or contact lenses may be worn during the test. If corrective lenses are needed to meet the vision standard, then they must be worn while driving.**

When using the Snellen test, the driver is positioned 20 feet from the wall chart; thus "20" is the numerator in the test results. The number of the last line of type the driver can read accurately is recorded as the denominator. If a test other than the Snellen is used, the test results should be recorded in Snellen-equivalent values.

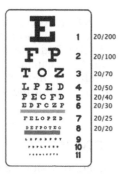

There are versions of the Snellen chart that compensate for failure to read letters because of limited English reading skill, not because of poor eyesight. One example is the "Snellen Eye Chart – Illiterate" that requires the individual to indicate the orientation of the letter "E" on the chart.

Peripheral vision

The requirement for peripheral vision is at least 70° in the horizontal meridian for each eye. Some form of "confrontational" testing is often used to evaluate peripheral vision. This involves the examiner sitting in front of the driver and asking the driver to indicate when he/she sees the examiner's finger out of the corner of his/her eyes. When test results are inconclusive, evaluation should be performed by a specialist with equipment capable of precise measurements.

Color vision

Drivers must be able to recognize and distinguish among red, amber, and green, the standard colors of traffic control signals and devices. True color perception is not required.

Additional evaluation

Eye trauma and eye-related disease can harm vision and interfere with safe driving. Some eye diseases are seen more frequently with increased age or are secondary to other diseases such as diabetes or atherosclerosis.

The DOT medical examiner may not be able to evaluate eye diseases adequately and may send the driver to an ophthalmologist or optometrist. The medical examiner would then consider the documented results and the specialist opinion when determining if the driver's vision meets qualification requirements.

Monocular Vision

Monocular vision occurs when the vision requirements are met in only one eye, with or without the aid of corrective lenses, regardless of cause or degree of vision loss in the other eye. In low illumination or glare, monocular vision causes deficiencies in contrast recognition and depth perception compared to binocular vision.

> **Monocular vision is disqualifying if the driver cannot qualify under the alternate vision standard in §391.44 and is otherwise medically qualified.**

Under the **alternate vision standard in §391.44,** on and after March 22, 2022, the driver is required to present to the medical examiner a Vision Evaluation Report (MCSA-5871) completed by an optometrist/opthalmologist in the 45 days prior to the date of the DOT exam. The medical examiner should review the

MCSA-5871 and complete all other aspects of the certification exam for a driver with monocular vision and determine if the driver is medically qualified for **no more than 1 year**.

For a driver previously qualified under a federal vision exemption or the federal vision waiver study Grandfather program (§391.64):

- The driver must qualify under the alternate vision standard no later than 11:59 P.M. on March 21, 2023.

- Medical cards issued under the federal vision exemption are not valid on and after March 22, 2023.

Federal Vision Exemption Program

The federal vision exemption program will not be used on and after March 22, 2022 due to the adoption of the alternate vision standard in 391.44. The FMCSA Vision Exemption Program was for drivers who lost vision in one eye (monocular vision), to allow them to operate a CMV in interstate commerce. The vision exemption was issued for a maximum of 2 years. The driver must have been otherwise medically qualified under §391.41(b)(1-13) or hold another valid medical exemption as needed. The driver must have obtained an annual medical exam and an eye exam by an ophthalmologist or an optometrist. The motor carrier is responsible for ensuring that the driver had the required documentation before driving a commercial vehicle. **The driver is responsible for carrying both the vision exemption and the medical examiner's certificate while driving and keeping both current not later than March 21, 2023, after which all medical cards issued under the federal vision exemption program are void.**

Qualified Under §391.64: "Grandfathered"

Before the start of the Federal Vision Exemption Program, the FMCSA conducted a vision study program that ran from 1992 to 1996. At the end of that study, 2,656 drivers received a one-time letter confirming participation in the study and granting a continued exemption from the vision requirement for as long as the driver was otherwise medically fit for duty and could meet the vision qualification requirements with the one eye.

Drivers under the grandfather program must qualify for the alternate vision standard no later than March 21, 2023 after which all medical cards under the grandfather program are void. A driver who was grandfathered must have had an annual medical exam and an eye exam by an ophthalmologist or optometrist. There are very few remaining drivers from that program. At the annual medical exam, the driver should present to the medical examiner the letter identifying the driver as a participant in the program and a copy of the eye specialist report. If recertified, the driver's medical card would indicate that the driver is "Qualified by operation of 49 CFR 391.64."

For more details, contact the Federal Vision Exemption Program:

- Phone: (703) 448-3094
- E-mail: medicalexemptions@dot.gov

Hearing

The standard: §391.41(b)(11)

A person is physically qualified to drive a commercial motor vehicle if that person:

- First perceives a forced whispered voice in the better ear from at least 5 feet away, with or without the use of a hearing aid; or

- If tested with an audiometric device, does not have an average hearing loss in the better ear greater than 40 decibels at 500 Hz, 1,000 Hz, and 2,000 Hz, with or without a hearing aid.

> The frequency range of hearing for a healthy young person is about 20 - 20,000 Hz.

 Key points:

- Two tests are used to screen hearing: a forced-whisper test and/or an audiometric test.

- The required tests screen for hearing loss in the range of normal conversational tones.

- Either test may be administered first. If the driver meets the hearing standard on the first test, the second test can be skipped.

- Both ears must be tested, but drivers must only pass one test in one ear to be considered qualified.

- When a hearing aid is used to pass the hearing test, the hearing aid must be used while driving.

- A driver is disqualified if he/she fails both the forced-whisper test AND the audiometric test.

STANDARDS

Public safety considerations:

- Hearing plays a role in safe driving. Hearing warning sounds, such as horns, train signals, and sirens may allow the driver to react to a potential hazard before it is visible. An auditory alarm or changes in the usual sound of the engine or vehicle carriage may be the first indication that the vehicle may require maintenance.

- Hearing loss can interfere with communication between the driver and other people such as dispatchers, loading dock personnel, passengers, and law enforcement officers.

- Balance is required for safe driving and task performance (e.g., vehicle inspections, securing loads) and when getting into, and out of, trucks and buses.

Medications:

Medications may be used to preserve hearing, reduce inflammatory disorders causing pain, and/or control dizziness causing loss of balance. The examiner must confirm that the agents are having the desired effect and whether there are any effects and/or side effects that interfere with safe driving (e.g., drug, food, and/or alcohol interactions, excessive drowsiness, or allergic reaction).

Agents used to treat:	include:
Acute vertigo	• Antihistaminic antiemetics, • Benzodiazepines, • Anticholinergics, and • Sympathomimetics.
Infections and inflammation of the external auditory canal	• Topical antibiotics, • Topical steroids, and • Topical antibiotic-steroid combinations.
Infections and inflammation of the middle ear (otitis media)	• Oral antibiotics, and • Oral steroids.

Hearing loss can be a symptom of a disease rather than a discrete disorder. In some cases, hearing loss may be treated and reversed.

Disqualifying conditions

The FMCSA's *Conference on Neurological Disorders and Commercial Drivers* report recommends disqualification when there is a diagnosis of:

- Meniere's disease,
- Labyrinthine fistula, or
- Non-functioning labyrinth.

Vertigo

Vertigo is generally caused by an inner-ear abnormality. Uncontrolled vertigo is disqualifying.

The *Conference on Neurological Disorders and Commercial Drivers* report recommends that the driver may be certified after completing at least 2 months symptom free with a diagnosis of:

- Benign positional vertigo, or
- Acute and chronic peripheral vestibulopathy.

Testing standards

Test	Standard
Forced whisper	The driver must first perceive a forced whispered voice in one ear at not less than 5 feet. A hearing aid may be used during the test. If the driver cannot pass the forced-whisper test with a hearing aid, referral to an audiologist, otolaryngologist, or hearing-aid center is required.
Audiometric	The driver must have an average hearing loss in one ear of no more than 40 dB. "Average" means the average of test results for 500 hertz (Hz), 1,000 Hz, and 2,000 Hz. When a hearing aid is to be worn during audiometric testing, an audiologist or hearing-aid center should perform the test using appropriate audiometric equipment.

VI. *Qualification Standards*

The audiometric test

The hearing requirement for an audiometric test is
based on hearing loss only at the 500 Hz, 1,000 Hz, and
2,000 Hz frequencies that are typical of normal conver-
sation. The readings for the three frequencies are aver-
aged for each ear. To pass, *one ear* must show an
average hearing loss that is less than or equal to 40 dB.

The test results are for an audiometer calibrated to the
American National Standards Institute (ANSI) Z24.5-
1951 standard. When an audiometer that is calibrated
to a different standard is used, the test results must be
converted to the ANSI standard. To convert International Organization for Standardization (ISO) test results to the ANSI standard, subtract from the ISO test
results:

- 14 dB for 500 Hz
- 10 dB for 1,000 Hz
- 8.5 dB for 2,000 Hz

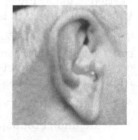

The forced-whisper test

The forced-whisper test is much
like it sounds: the examiner whispers to the driver from a distance
of 5 feet to the side or behind the
driver, testing one ear at a time using a sequence of
words, numbers, or letters. The examiner asks the
driver to repeat the whispered sequence; to pass, the
driver must respond correctly.

The whisper test is completed for both ears even if the
initial test result meets the hearing requirement.

A hearing aid may be worn while testing.

➤ **When a hearing aid is used to qualify, the
hearing aid must be worn while driving.**

Additional tests

Ear trauma and disease can affect hearing and/or balance and interfere with safe driving and non-driving tasks. When findings are inconclusive, additional tests and/or additional evaluation by a specialist – usually an audiologist or otolaryngologist – may be required to obtain enough medical information to determine certification status.

Hearing aids

A driver who uses a hearing aid to qualify must wear a hearing aid while driving. The examiner has to mark the "wearing hearing aid" checkbox on both the Medical Examination Report form and the medical examiner's certificate.

It is *recommended* that drivers who need to use a hearing aid should carry a spare power source for the hearing aid. Without a backup power source, the driver may be cited for driving while physically unqualified if the primary power source fails.

STANDARDS

135

Hypertension

The standard: §391.41(b)(6)

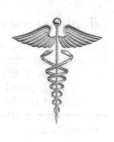

A person is physically qualified to drive a commercial motor vehicle (CMV) if that person has no current clinical diagnosis of high blood pressure (BP) likely to interfere with his/her ability to operate a CMV safely.

 Key points:

- If a driver has hypertension and/or is being medicated for hypertension, he or she should be recertified more frequently (at least annually) or may even be disqualified.

- The FMCSA identifies three stages of hypertension:
  - Stage 1 (140/90-159/99): Driver may be certified for 1 year.
  - Stage 2 (160/100-179/109): Driver may be certified one time for 3 months.
  - Stage 3 (greater than 180/110): Driver is disqualified.

- Nearly one-third of the adult population has hypertension, and about one-fourth of them are unaware they have it.

- Lifestyle changes and drug treatment can be effective at reducing hypertension.

Public safety considerations:

According to national surveys, 29 percent of all U.S. adults 18 years and older have blood pressure greater than or equal to 140/90 or are taking medication for hypertension. The prevalence of hypertension is nearly equal for men and women. Among adults with hypertension:

- 78% are aware of their condition,

- 68% are treated with antihypertensive medication, and

- 64% achieve BP less than 140/90 with treatment.

Hypertension alone is unlikely to cause sudden collapse; however, hypertension can lead to the development of more serious cardiovascular disease, peripheral vascular disease, and chronic renal insufficiency. A BP greater than or equal to 140/90 is deemed high for most individuals without other significant cardiovascular risk factors.

In individuals ranging from 40 to 89 years of age, for every 20 mm Hg systolic or 10 mm Hg diastolic increase in BP, there is a doubling of mortality from both heart disease and stroke. The relationship between BP and risk of cardiovascular disease is continuous, consistent, and independent of other risk factors. Both elevated systolic and diastolic BP are risk factors for coronary heart disease.

STANDARDS

Drivers are at greater risk

Once in the profession, CMV drivers have a greater propensity to develop hypertension than their peers in other professions. Studies have shown that the percentage of drivers with hypertension increases:

- From 29% in drivers with fewer than 10 years of driving experience,

- To 32% in drivers with 10-20 years of experience, and

- To 39% in drivers with more than 20 years of driving experience.

As the years of experience rise, part of the increase in hypertension may relate to accompanying aging, increase in body mass, or decline in physical activity.

Treatment reduces risk

Drivers can reduce the risks of high blood pressure. Lifestyle changes and drug treatment can be effective at reducing hypertension, thereby reducing the risk of cardiovascular problems or even death. Studies have found that antihypertensive therapy reduces the incidence of stroke, heart attack, and heart failure.

Contemporary medical therapies are effective in lowering BP, reducing complications, and are generally regarded as safe.

The examiner's role

The medical examiner's fundamental obligation is to establish whether a driver has high BP that is likely to interfere with the ability to operate a CMV safely, thus endangering public safety.

The examination is based on:

- Information provided by the driver (i.e., the health history);

- Objective data found through measuring blood pressure and conducting a physical exam; and

- Additional testing requested by the medical examiner.

The examiner's assessment should consider physical, psychological, and environmental factors affecting BP.

Physical exam:

The examiner must:

- Measure the driver's BP;

- Confirm BP greater than 139/89 with a second measurement taken later during the exam; and

- Check pulse rate, strength, and rhythm.

? Q: Can the examiner's assistant(s) take the BP readings?
A: Yes, under the supervision of the examiner; however, the FMCSA recommends that the examiner personally confirm the BP if it's disqualifying.

If a driver uses medication to control hypertension, the driver is still considered to have a diagnosis of hypertension. When antihypertensive medication is used to treat an underlying condition other than high BP, certification is based on the underlying condition and tolerance to the medication.

Confirming an elevated BP

A BP higher than or equal to 140/90 should be confirmed with a second measurement taken later during the exam. A driver's BP, especially systolic pressure, will fluctuate in a short time from normal to elevated and back to normal as a response to many factors, including:

- Circadian cycle;

- Emotional and physical states;

- Transient hypertension (e.g., "white coat syndrome");

- Use of left versus right arm during BP measurement; and

- Problems with technique, such as:

  - Placing the BP cuff over clothing instead of on the skin,

  - Using an inappropriately-sized BP cuff, or

  - Positioning the arm incorrectly.

> A driver who is disqualified for high BP or uncontrolled hypertension should not be considered for recertification until the BP is stabilized at less than or equal to 140/90. Treatment should be well tolerated before considering certifying a driver with a history of Stage 3 hypertension.

Drivers with essential hypertension

"Essential" hypertension, also known as primary hypertension, is the "usual" kind of high blood pressure, with no clear cause. It is thought to be linked to genetics, diet, obesity, and lack of exercise.

If a driver's essential hypertension is below Stage 1, the driver may be fully certified if all certification criteria are met. The examiner may evaluate the driver for signs of cardiovascular disease and target organ damage, which may affect certification.

When a driver's essential BP is in the range of Stage 1 or Stage 2 hypertension, the medical examiner is to consider these additional factors:

- Type of examination (certification or recertification);

- Current certification interval (1-2 years or 3 months);

- Treatment (lifestyle changes, use of medication); and

- Severity of hypertension prior to treatment (particularly if there is a history of Stage 3 hypertension).

The purpose of a one-time, three-month certificate is to allow a driver with high BP to drive while taking steps to lower the elevated BP. It is not meant as a means to indefinitely extend driving privileges for a driver with a condition that is associated with long-term risks. **NOTE:** "One-time" means the examiner cannot issue consecutive three-month certificates for BP greater than 140/90. It does not mean once in a lifetime.

For a driver with high BP or hypertension to maintain continuous certification, the driver must demonstrate, during the exam, a BP at or less than 140/90.

Drivers with secondary hypertension

"Secondary" hypertension is high blood pressure caused by another, known medical condition.

The prevalence of secondary hypertension in the general population is estimated at between 5% and 20%. The examiner will seek to obtain information that assesses the underlying cause, the effectiveness of treatment, and any side effects that may interfere with driving.

If the secondary hypertension IS NOT treated through surgery, the guidelines for essential hypertension are to be followed.

If the secondary hypertension IS treated through surgery:

• A decision on DOT certification should not be made until at least three months after the surgery.

• The maximum certification period is one year, followed by annual recertification exams.

• The FMCSA's recommendation is to certify drivers whose BP is below Stage 1, but disqualification is an option if the examiner believes the driver's overall medical condition endangers health and safety.

• The examiner may order additional tests and/or consultation as needed.

141

Stage 1 Hypertension

BP = At least 140/90 but less than 160/100

Stage 1 hypertension is usually symptom-free, and blood pressure (BP) in this range is considered a low risk for hypertension-related incapacitation. However, all hypertensive drivers should be strongly encouraged to consult with a primary care provider to ensure appropriate therapy and healthcare education.

Certification recommendations

IF:	THEN the driver should be:
It is the first exam at which the driver has BP equivalent to Stage 1 hypertension and the driver: • Has no history of hypertension, and • Does not use antihypertensive medication to control BP	certified for 1 year.
1. The driver was issued a one-year certificate for untreated Stage 1 hypertension and has not been prescribed drugs to control high BP (i.e., a hypertensive driver is asking to be recertified after getting a one-year certificate); or 2. The driver has a diagnosis of hypertension treated with medication and tolerates treatment with no side effects that interfere with driving (this applies to a driver with inadequately controlled BP) NOTE: The driver should be advised that failure to lower BP to less than or equal to 140/90 will render the driver medically unqualified after the 3 months expire.	certified for 3 months.
The driver has: • A one-time, 3-month certificate for elevated BP or hypertension and BP greater than 140/90; • A history of Stage 3 hypertension and BP greater than 140/90; or • BP greater than or equal to 180/110, regardless of any other considerations	disqualified.
The driver was disqualified for Stage 1 hypertension and has lowered his or her BP to less than 140/90	recertified for 1 year.

Certification recommendations, Continued

IF:	THEN the driver should be:
The driver was disqualified for Stage 3 hypertension, has lowered his or her BP to less than 140/90, and tolerates medications	recertified for 6 months.

NOTE: "One-time" means the driver cannot receive consecutive 3-month certificates for BP greater than 140/90. It does not mean once in a lifetime.

Follow-up: A driver with elevated BP or hypertension should have at least an annual medical exam.

When certified for three months, the driver should seek drug therapy to lower BP to less than or equal to 140/90 to be recertified at the follow-up exam.

Stage 2 Hypertension

BP = At least 160/100 but less than 180/110

A driver with Stage 2 hypertension should seek drug therapy to lower blood pressure. Effective BP management includes routine primary provider follow-up and periodic screens for the presence of target organ damage and signs of cardiovascular disease.

➤ **A driver with Stage 2 hypertension should only be certified one time for 3 months.**

Certification recommendations

IF:	THEN the driver should be:
• It is the first exam at which the driver has BP equivalent to Stage 2 hypertension, and • The driver has no history of hypertension and does not use medication to control BP	certified for 3 months.*

143

Certification recommendations, Continued

IF:	THEN the driver should be:
• The driver has a diagnosis of hypertension treated with medication, and • The driver tolerates treatment with no side effects that interfere with driving	certified for 3 months.*
• The driver currently holds a one-time, 3-month certificate for Stage 2 hypertension and BP is greater than 140/90; • The driver has a history of Stage 3 hypertension and BP is greater than 140/90; or • The driver's BP is greater than or equal to 180/110, regardless of any other considerations	not certified.

*A driver issued a one-time, 3-month certificate should be advised that:

• To qualify at follow-up, BP should be at or less than 140/90.

• If the driver qualifies at follow-up, an entirely new medical exam will be required before a new, 1-year certificate will be issued.

• If the driver fails to lower BP by the expiration date of the one-time, 3-month certificate, the driver will be disqualified until BP is at or less than 140/90 at examination.

NOTE: "One-time" means the driver cannot receive consecutive 3-month certificates for BP greater than 140/90. It does not mean once in a lifetime.

Provided treatment is well tolerated and the driver demonstrates BP of 140/90 or less, the driver may be certified for 1 year from the date of the follow-up examination.

Follow-up: The driver must have a follow-up exam on or before the 3-month certificate expires. If the driver has BP less than or equal to 140/90, the driver may be certified for 1 year.

NOTE: Unlike in the past, the expiration date of a medical certificate cannot be "extended." A driver issued a 3-month certificate must have an entirely new examination and – if certified – be issued an entirely new certificate at the follow-up exam. If issued a 1-year certificate at follow-up, that certificate will expire 12 months after the follow-up exam.

If a certification decision cannot be made and the exam result is placed into "Determination Pending" status (for up to 45 days, so the examiner can gather more information before making a decision), then a new certificate will not be issued at the time of the exam and the driver must rely on his or her *existing* medical card to continue driving. If a certification decision is made before the end of the 45-day period, the expiration date of the new certificate (if one is issued) will be based on the date of the certification decision, not the date of the exam.

Stage 3 Hypertension

BP = At least 180 / 110

Stage 3 hypertension carries a high risk for the development of acute hypertension-related symptoms that could impair judgment and driving ability. Results of elevated blood pressure (BP) can include sudden stroke, acute pulmonary edema, subarachnoid hemorrhage, aortic dissection, or aortic aneurysm rupture.

➤ **Drivers with Stage 3 hypertension should not be certified.**

Meningismus, acute neurological deficits, abrupt onset of shortness of breath, or severe, ripping back or chest pain could signal an impending hypertensive catastrophe that requires immediate cessation of driving and emergency medical care. Symptoms of hypertensive urgency such as headache and nausea are likely to be

145

more subtle in onset and more amenable to treatment than a hypertensive emergency.

Certification recommendations

IF:	THEN the driver should be:
The driver has Stage 3 hypertension	disqualified and advised to seek (or should be provided) immediate medical attention.
The driver has a history of Stage 3 hypertension but at examination has BP at or less than 140/90 and treatment that is well tolerated	considered for 6-month certification.
The driver is receiving semi-annual exams due to a history of Stage 3 hypertension, but at the current exam his or her BP is equivalent to Stage 1 or Stage 2 hypertension	given a one-time, 3-month certificate in accordance with Stage 1 or Stage 2 hypertension guidelines, as determined on a case-by-case basis.

A driver with a history of Stage 3 hypertension should only be certified for a maximum of 6 months at a time.

If the examiner believes that a BP greater than 140/90 at rest indicates an unacceptable risk for development of Stage 3 hypertension and the onset of hypertension-related symptoms, then he or she may temporarily disqualify the driver until BP is at or less than 140/90 and treatment is well tolerated.

For example, when maximum doses of multiple antihypertensive medications fail to bring BP down below 140/90, a more aggressive treatment plan should be monitored for effectiveness, interactions, and tolerance prior to driver certification.

> At follow-up, the driver should have a medical exam at least every 6 months.

Cardiovascular

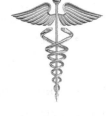

The standard: §391.41(b)(4)

A person is physically qualified to drive a commercial motor vehicle (CMV) if that person has no current clinical diagnosis of myocardial infarction (heart attack), angina pectoris (chest pain), coronary insufficiency, thrombosis (clotting in a blood vessel), or any other cardiovascular disease (CVD) of a variety known to be accompanied by syncope (fainting), dyspnea (shortness of breath), collapse, or congestive cardiac failure.

 Key points:

- Numerous cardiovascular diseases may lead to shortened certification periods or even disqualification.

- Among the conditions/devices that are disqualifying:
  - Implantable cardioverter-defibrillators;
  - Implantable cardiac defibrillator/pacemaker combination devices;
  - Thoracic aneurysms greater than 3.5 cm in size;
  - An untreated aneurysm;
  - An abdominal aortic aneurysm greater than 5 cm in size;
  - Untreated deep-vein thrombosis;
  - Pain at rest from peripheral vascular disease or intermittent claudication;
  - Unstable angina (chest pain);
  - Hypertrophic or restrictive cardiomyopathy; or
  - Heart conditions that cause fainting.

- Refer to the Cardiovascular Recommendation Tables (see "Online Resources" in Chapter 9).
- Refer also to the *Cardiovascular Advisory Panel Guidelines for the Medical Examination of Commercial Motor Vehicle Drivers:*

Public safety considerations:

The fundamental question when deciding if a commercial driver should be medically certified is whether the driver has a CVD that increases the risk of sudden death or incapacitation and creates a danger to the safety and health of the driver, as well as the public.

A number of concerns predispose commercial drivers to an increased risk of CVD:

- The average driver age is 39 years (as of 2009).

- Obesity and a sedentary lifestyle increase the risk of CVD. Both are more common in the commercial driving population than in the general population.

- Driving stressors, such as traffic congestion, erratic shift work, a sense of responsibility for others, and emotional distress due to belligerent passengers, can lead to the release of certain chemicals that increase the likelihood of changes in arterial tone, heart function, and tendency for blood clots, particularly given the aging workforce in the United States.

- Drivers are exposed to other environmental stressors that may be detrimental to the cardiovascular system, such as excessive noise, temperature extremes, air pollution, and vibration.

The major clinical manifestations of CVD are heart attack, chest pain, sudden death, and congestive heart failure. An irregular heartbeat (arrhythmia) is the most likely cause of sudden driver incapacitation. However, coronary heart disease (CHD) is the most common cause. Coronary heart disease frequently presents itself as a heart attack (50%), chest pain (30%), and sudden death (20%). Sudden cardiac dysfunction is particularly relevant to safety-sensitive positions like driving.

The effect of heart disease on driving must be viewed in relation to the general health of the driver. Other medical conditions may worsen a cardiovascular condition, so certification depends on a comprehensive assessment of overall health.

Disqualification requires that the CMV driver exhibit a higher-than-acceptable likelihood of being incapacitated due to a cardiac event, resulting in an increased risk to the safety and health of the driver and the public.

The exam:

During the physical exam, the examiner is expected to ask the same questions that would be asked of any individual being assessed for cardiovascular concerns. In addition to questions and checklists on the Medical Examination Report form, the examiner should ask about and document cardiovascular symptoms.

The examiner should check for:

• Murmurs, extra heart sounds, or irregular heartbeat (arrhythmia);

• An enlarged heart; and

• Abnormal pulse and amplitude, carotid or arterial bruits, or varicose veins.

The examiner must document any discussion with the driver about history, medication, and abnormal findings concerning the cardiovascular system.

Aneurysms and Blood Vessel/Vein Diseases

1. Abdominal Aortic Aneurysm

An aneurysm is a bulge or "ballooning" in the wall of an artery. The majority of abdominal aortic aneurysms (AAAs) occur in the sixth and seventh decades of life and occur more frequently in males than in females by a 3:1 ratio. The majority of AAAs are asymptomatic. An AAA can be associated with other cardiovascular disease.

The overall detection rate of AAAs on examination is 31%. Detection during a physical exam depends on aneurysm size and is affected by obesity.

Rupture is the most serious complication of an AAA and can be life threatening. The risk of rupture increases as the aneurysm increases in size.

Size	Rate of Rupture
< 4 cm	Rarely ruptures.
< 5 cm	1% to 3% per year.
5-6 cm	5% to 10% per year.
> 7 cm	Approximately 20% per year.

Monitoring of an aneurysm is advised because the growth rate can vary and rapid expansion can occur.

Aneurysms can be surgically repaired to prevent rupture. The decision by the treating provider not to surgically repair an aneurysm does not mean that the driver can be certified to drive safely. However, a recommendation to surgically repair an aneurysm disqualifies the driver until the aneurysm has been repaired and a satisfactory recovery period has passed.

Waiting period before certification: At least 3 months after surgical repair of an aneurysm.

Maximum certification period: 1 year

Certification recommendation:

 <u>Certify</u> if:
- The AAA is less than 4 cm and the driver is asymptomatic (does not show symptoms); or
- The AAA is 4-5 cm and the driver is asymptomatic and has clearance from a cardiovascular specialist who understands the demands of commercial driving; or
- The AAA is surgically repaired and the driver meets the guidelines for post-surgical repair of aneurysms.

✗ <u>Do not certify</u> if:
- The driver has symptoms, regardless of AAA size; or
- The driver received a recommendation for surgical repair, regardless of AAA size, from a cardiovascular specialist who understands the demands of commercial driving; or
- The AAA is 4-5 cm and driver does not have medical clearance for commercial driving from a cardiovascular specialist; or
- The AAA is greater than or equal to 5 cm; or
- The AAA has increased more than 0.5 cm during a 6-month period, regardless of size.

Monitoring/testing: Ultrasound is recommended to monitor change in size. When post-surgical treatment includes anticoagulant therapy, the driver should meet monitoring guidelines.

Follow-up: Annual medical exams.

Anticoagulant Therapy

Medications to prevent blood clots may be used in the treatment of cardiovascular or neurological conditions. The certification decision should be based on the underlying medical disease or disorder, not the medication itself. The most current guidelines for the use of warfarin (Coumadin) for cardiovascular diseases are found in the *Cardiovascular Advisory Panel Guidelines for the Medical Examination of Commercial Motor Vehicle Drivers* (see "Online Resources" in Chapter 9).

For a cardiovascular condition:

Waiting period before certification: At least 1 month stabilized

Maximum certification period: 1 year

Certification recommendation:

 Certify if the driver:
- Is stabilized on medication for at least 1 month,
- Provides a copy of the international normalized ratio (INR)* results at the exam, and
- Has at least monthly INR monitoring.

✗ Do not certify if:
- INR is not being monitored,
- INR is not therapeutic, or
- The underlying disease is disqualifying.

*The International Normalized Ratio (INR) is a measure of the ability of blood to clot.

Monitoring/testing: The driver should obtain INR monitoring at least monthly.

Follow-up: The driver should bring results of INR monitoring to the exam.

For a neurological condition:

The driver should not be certified if he/she has a cerebrovascular disorder, due to the high rate of complications associated with bleeding that can incapacitate the driver while operating a vehicle.

2. Acute Deep Vein Thrombosis

Commercial drivers are at an increased risk for developing acute deep vein thrombosis (DVT) – blood clots – due to long hours of sitting. DVT can be the source of pulmonary emboli that can cause gradual or sudden incapacitation or death. Adequate treatment with anticoagulants decreases the risk of recurrent thrombosis by approximately 80%.

Waiting period before certification: As needed until the cause is confirmed and treatment is adequate, effective, safe, and stable.

Maximum certification period: 1 year

Certification recommendation:

✓ Certify if the driver has no lasting, acute DVT.

✗ Do not certify if the driver's DVT is not effectively treated.

Monitoring/testing: When DVT treatment includes anticoagulant therapy, the driver should meet monitoring guidelines for that therapy (see above).

Follow-up: Annual medical exam.

3. Chronic Thrombotic Venous Disease

Chronic thrombotic venous disease of the legs increases the risk of pulmonary emboli (clots or other obstructions in a blood vessel); however, there is insufficient research to confirm the level of risk. The medical examiner must evaluate on a case-by-case basis to determine if the driver meets cardiovascular requirements.

Waiting period before certification: As needed until the cause is confirmed and treatment is adequate, effective, safe, and stable.

Maximum certification period: 2 years

Certification recommendation:

 Certify if the driver has no symptoms of the disease.

Follow-up: Biennial medical exam (every 2 years).

4. Intermittent Claudication

Approximately 7-9% of persons with peripheral vascular disease develop intermittent claudication – a painful circulatory condition that causes cramping and limping – the primary symptom of obstructive vascular disease of the lower extremity. In severe cases, tissue death, nervous-system disorders, and atrophy may occur.

Waiting period before certification: At least 3 months after surgical repair, and at least until the cause is confirmed and treatment is adequate, effective, safe, and stable.

Maximum certification: 1 year

Certification recommendation:

✓ Certify after surgery if the driver has relief of symptoms and no other disqualifying cardiovascular disease.

✗ Do not certify if the driver has pain at rest.

Follow-up: Annual medical exams.

5. Other Aneurysms

Aneurysms – bulges in artery walls – can develop in visceral and peripheral arteries and venous vessels. Rupture of any of these aneurysms can lead to gradual or sudden incapacitation and death. Much of the information on aortic aneurysms is applicable to aneurysms in other arteries.

Waiting period before certification: At least 3 months after surgery.

Maximum certification: 1 year

Certification recommendation:

 Certify if the driver has:
  • Effective surgical repair of the aneurysm, and

  • Clearance from a cardiovascular specialist who understands the demands of commercial driving.

Follow-up: Annual medical exams.

6. Peripheral Vascular Disease

Obstructive vascular disease of the lower extremities is a widely recognized peripheral vascular disease (PVD) in adults. PVD is usually a slow, progressive disease with a benign course that carries little to no risk for gradual or sudden incapacitation.

For the driver, pain at rest represents a critical degree of ischemia (inadequate blood supply) and is disqualifying because of the likelihood of reduced dexterity in the affected limb. PVD may require surgical repair or amputation.

Waiting period before certification: At least 3 months after surgery.

Maximum certification: 1 year

Certification recommendation:

✓ Certify if the driver has no other disqualifying cardiovascular disease.

✗ Do not certify if the driver has pain at rest.

Follow-up: Annual medical exams.

7. Pulmonary Emboli

Deep vein thrombosis (clotting) can be one of the sources of pulmonary emboli (PE), a mass that blocks a blood vessel. PE can cause gradual or sudden incapacitation and significant morbidity and mortality.

Waiting period before certification: At least 3 months with no PE

Maximum certification: 1 year

Certification recommendation:

✓ Certify if the driver has:
  • Appropriate long-term treatment, and
  • No other disqualifying cardiovascular disease.

✗ Do not certify if the driver has symptoms.

Monitoring/testing: When PE treatment includes anticoagulant therapy, the driver should meet monitoring guidelines for that therapy (see above).

Follow-up: Annual medical exams.

8. Superficial Phlebitis

Although superficial phlebitis (inflammation of a vein wall) is a benign and self-limited disease, deep vein thrombosis (clotting) is often a coexisting condition and needs to be excluded during the course of examination.

Waiting period before certification: The driver should not be certified until the cause is confirmed and treatment is adequate, effective, safe, and stable.

Maximum certification period: 2 years

Certification recommendation:

✓ <u>Certify</u> if the driver is otherwise medically qualified.

✗ <u>Do not certify</u> if the driver has coexisting deep vein thrombosis (DVT) and does not meet the DVT guidelines (see above).

Follow-up: Biennial medical exams (every 2 years).

9. Thoracic Aneurysm

While relatively rare, a thoracic aneurysm (a weakened and bulging area in the upper part of the aorta) are increasing in frequency. The size of the aorta is considered the major factor in determining risk for dissection or rupture of a thoracic aneurysm.

Waiting period before certification: At least 3 months after surgery

Maximum certification: 1 year

Certification recommendation:

 <u>Certify</u> if the driver has:
  • A thoracic aneurysm less than 3.5 cm; or

  • A surgically repaired thoracic aneurysm and the driver meets post-surgical repair of aneurysm guidelines, including:
    – Has completed surgical repair waiting period, and

    – Has medical clearance from a cardiovascular specialist who understands the demands of commercial driving.

157

<u>Do not certify</u> if the driver has a thoracic aneurysm greater than 3.5 cm.

Follow-up: Annual medical exams.

10. Varicose Veins

Varicose veins with the associated symptoms and complications affect more than 20 million people in the United States. Complications include chronic venous insufficiency, leg ulcerations, and recurrent deep-vein clotting.

The presence of varicose veins does not medically disqualify a commercial driver.

Waiting period before certification: As needed until the cause is confirmed and treatment is adequate, effective, safe, and stable.

Maximum certification period: 2 years

Certification recommendation:

<u>Certify</u> if the driver has no complications.

Follow-up: Biennial medical exams (every 2 years).

Cardiac Arrhythmias

The majority of sudden cardiac deaths are thought to be secondary to ventricular tachycardia (an abnormally fast heartbeat) or ventricular fibrillation (an irregular heartbeat) and occur most often when there is no prior diagnosis of heart disease.

Determining risk is difficult because of the numerous variables that have to be considered. The prognosis is generally determined by the underlying heart disease. While defibrillation may restore a normal rhythm, there remains a high risk of recurrence.

When a driver has a history of arrhythmia or uses an anti-arrhythmia device, the medical examiner should consider the following:

- Is the underlying heart disease disqualifying?

- What is the risk for sudden death?

- What is the risk for cerebral hypoperfusion (reduced blood flow to the brain) and loss of consciousness?

1. Implantable Cardioverter-Defibrillators

Implantable cardioverter-defibrillators (ICD) are electronic devices that treat cardiac arrest, ventricular fibrillation, and ventricular tachycardia through the delivery of rapid-paced stimuli or shock therapy.

ICDs treat but do not prevent arrhythmias. Therefore, the driver remains at risk for loss of consciousness. The management of the underlying disease is not effective enough for the driver to be certified. Combination ICD/pacemaker devices are also ineffective in preventing incapacitating cardiac arrhythmia events.

Certification recommendation:

✗ Do not certify if the driver has an ICD or ICD/pacemaker combination device.

See also: The Implantable Defibrillator Recommendation Table in the *Cardiovascular Advisory Panel Guidelines for the Medical Examination of Commercial Motor Vehicle Drivers* (see "Online Resources" in Chapter 9)

2. Pacemakers

A pacemaker is an implantable device designed to treat bradycardia (slowness of the heart). When assessing the risk for sudden, unexpected incapacitation in a driver with a pacemaker, the underlying disease must be considered.

Both sinus node dysfunction and atrioventricular block have variable long-term prognoses, depending on the underlying disease.

Reduced blood flow to the brain (cerebral hypoperfusion) is usually corrected by support of heart rate through the implantation of a pacemaker.

Currently, pacemakers and the lead systems are reliable and durable over the long term.

Waiting period before certification:

Underlying disease	Waiting period after pacemaker implantation
• Sinus node dysfunction, or • Atrioventricular block	At least 1 month
• Neurocardiogenic syncope, or • Hypersensitive carotid sinus with syncope	At least 3 months

Maximum certification period: 1 year

Certification recommendation:

 Certify if the driver has:
  • Documentation indicating the presence of a functioning pacemaker,

  • Documentation indicating completion of routine pacemaker checks, and

  • No disqualifying underlying disease.

✗ Do not certify if the driver has:
  • An implantable cardiac defibrillator/pacemaker combination device, or

  • A disqualifying underlying disease.

Monitoring/testing: The driver should:

• Comply with scheduled function checks for the pacemaker, and

- Provide documentation of pacemaker function checks at the examination.

Follow-up: Annual medical exams.

See also: The Pacemaker Recommendation Table in the *Cardiovascular Advisory Panel Guidelines for the Medical Examination of Commercial Motor Vehicle Drivers* (see "Online Resources" in Chapter 9).

3. Supraventricular Arrhythmias

Supraventricular arrhythmias (irregular heartbeat originating above the lower heart) fall into two main categories: supraventricular tachycardia (SVT) and atrial fibrillation.

Supraventricular tachycardia — SVT is a common arrhythmia (heartbeat irregularity) that is usually not considered a risk for sudden death. On occasion, SVT can cause loss of consciousness or compromise cerebral function. The condition can be largely cured through catheter ablation, usually allowing drug therapy to be withdrawn.

Atrial fibrillation — The major risk associated with atrial fibrillation – a fast and irregular heartbeat – is the presence of an embolus (typically a blood clot) which can cause a stroke. Anticoagulants decrease the risk of stroke.

See the Supraventricular Tachycardias Recommendation Table for diagnosis-specific recommendations, as found in the *Cardiovascular Advisory Panel Guidelines for the Medical Examination of Commercial Motor Vehicle Drivers* (see "Online Resources" in Chapter 9).

The following are general recommendations.

Waiting period before certification: At least 1 month if anticoagulated adequately and the diagnosis is atrial fibrillation as the cause of stroke or risk for stroke, and following thoracic surgery.

STANDARDS

VI. Qualification Standards

At least 1 month after isthmus ablation and the diagnosis is atrial flutter.

At least 1 month if asymptomatic/treated asymptomatic and the diagnosis is:

- Atrioventricular nodal reentrant tachycardia,
- Atrioventricular reentrant tachycardia and Wolff-Parkinson-White syndrome,
- Atrial tachycardia, or
- Junctional tachycardia.

Maximum certification period: 1 year

Certification recommendations:

 Certify if the driver has:
- A controlled heart rate,
- Treatment for prevention of emboli that is effective and tolerated,
- No underlying disqualifying disease, and
- Clearance from a cardiovascular specialist who understands the demands of commercial driving.

X Do not certify if the condition causes:
- Loss of consciousness,
- Compromised cerebral function, or
- Sudden death resuscitation.

Monitoring/testing: The driver should:

- Comply with anticoagulant therapy guidelines (see previous sidebar), when appropriate; and
- Have annual evaluation by a cardiovascular specialist who understands the demands of commercial driving.

Follow-up: Annual medical exams.

Note: There are times when the medical assessment and the guidelines may yield different conclusions about the severity of the condition. A driver could have a benign underlying medical problem with an excellent prognosis but still not be medically qualified as a commercial driver. For example, if a benign supraventricular arrhythmia causes fainting, the driver cannot be medically certified until the problem has been corrected.

4. Ventricular Arrhythmias

Ventricular arrhythmias (irregular heartbeat originating in the lower heart) are categorized as ventricular fibrillation and ventricular tachycardia and are responsible for the majority of instances of cardiac-related sudden death. Most cases are caused by coronary heart disease, but can also occur in people with hearts that are structurally normal.

Certification parameters include:

• Left ventricular ejection fraction (LVEF, the amount of blood expelled when the heart contracts),

• Non-sustained ventricular tachycardia (NSVT), and

• Ventricular tachycardia (VT, a rapid heartbeat that starts in the ventricles).

Waiting period before certification: At least 1 month after drug or other therapy and the diagnosis is:

• Coronary heart disease,

• Right ventricular outflow VT, or

• Left ventricular VT from an unknown cause (idiopathic).

Maximum certification period: 1 year

Certification recommendations:

 Certify if the driver:
- Is not showing any symptoms;
- Has an identified, non-disqualifying, cardiac cause; and
- Has clearance from a cardiovascular specialist who understands the demands of commercial driving.

✗ Do not certify if the driver:
- Is showing symptoms;
- Has sustained VT;
- Has NSVT, LVEF less than 0.40 or 40%; or
- Has a diagnosis of hypertrophic cardiomyopathy, long QT interval syndrome, or Brugada syndrome.

Monitoring/testing: The driver should have an annual evaluation by a cardiovascular specialist who understands the demands of commercial driving.

Follow-up: Annual medical exams.

See also: The Ventricular Arrhythmias Recommendation Table in the *Cardiovascular Advisory Panel Guidelines for the Medical Examination of Commercial Motor Vehicle Drivers* (see "Online Resources" in Chapter 9).

Cardiovascular Tests

Detection of an undiagnosed heart or vascular finding during a physical exam may indicate the need for further testing before the driver can be certified. Diagnostic-specific testing may be required to detect the presence and/or severity of cardiovascular diseases. The additional testing may be ordered by the medical examiner, primary care physician, cardiologist, or cardiovascular surgeon.

The specialist must understand the role and function of a commercial driver. It is recommended that the DOT examiner include a description of the role of the driver and a copy of the applicable medical standard(s) and guidelines with the request.

Any additional tests should be recorded on the Medical Examination Report form under the TESTING section, and/or by attaching additional test reports.

Other testing if indicated

ETT - stress test results attached

Echocardiography

Echocardiography, which creates an image of the heart using ultrasound, can be used to assess left ventricular ejection fraction (LVEF), a measure of blood being pumped into the aorta. Echocardiography offers superior sensitivity and specificity compared to the standard exercise tolerance test (ETT) and is recommended after an abnormal resting electrocardiogram or non-diagnostic standard ETT.

The driver should have:

- An LVEF greater than or equal to 40%, and
- No pulmonary hypertension.

NOTE:

- Pulmonary hypertension is pulmonary artery pressure greater than 50% of systemic systolic blood as determined by echocardiography or cardiac catheterization.

- If echocardiography test results are inconclusive, some form of radionuclide imaging may be used to obtain the ejection fraction measurement.

Exercise Tolerance Test

The exercise tolerance test is the most common test used to evaluate workload capacity and detect cardiac abnormalities. The driver should be able to:

- Exercise to a workload capacity greater than 6 Metabolic Equivalents (METs) (see table below);

- Attain a heart rate greater than or equal to 85% of predicted maximum (unless on beta blockers);

- Have a rise in systolic blood pressure greater than or equal to 20 mm Hg without angina; and

- Have no significant ST segment depression.

METs chart

Activity	Example	METs required
Sedentary activity	Sitting, slow walking, and lifting light objects of no more than 10 pounds.	< 2
Light work	Carrying lightweight objects of no more than 20 pounds.	2 - 4
Medium work	Carrying moderate weight objects of up to 50 pounds.	4 - 6
Heavy and very heavy work	Carrying heavy objects and climbing stairs rapidly.	> 6

Remember: Medical fitness for duty includes the ability to perform strenuous work. Overall requirements for commercial drivers in general, along with the specific requirements in the driver's job description, are deciding factors in the certification process.

Coronary Heart Diseases

The major clinical manifestations of coronary heart disease (CHD) are:

- Acute myocardial infarction (heart attack);

- Angina pectoris (chest pain, either stable or unstable);

- Congestive heart failure; and

- Sudden death.

Sudden death occurs when an individual goes from a usual state of health to death within one hour. In some cases, those who suffer sudden death show no symptoms beforehand.

The incidence of crashes caused by sudden death is relatively low, primarily because of the length of time between the onset of the cardiovascular event and the incapacitation of the driver. Therefore, affected drivers should be educated about the warning signs of an impending CHD event, emphasizing that drivers may have only a short time following the onset of symptoms to safely stop the vehicle and call for medical assistance.

Predicting CHD

The major predictor of CHD is left ventricular function. Other indicators to be considered include general heath, age, arrhythmias, chest pain, associated vascular disease, and severity of CHD.

General recommendations

A qualified driver with CHD should:

- Obtain clearance from a cardiovascular specialist who understands the demands of commercial driving; and

167

- Tolerate cardiovascular medication and be:

  - Knowledgeable about medications used while driving,

  - Free from side effects that compromise driving ability, and

  - Compliant with the ongoing treatment plan.

1. Acute Myocardial Infarction

The first few months following an acute myocardial infarction (MI) – a heart attack – pose the greatest risk of death, with most such deaths occurring suddenly. Current opinion among clinicians is that post-MI drivers may safely return to any job-related task as long as there is no exercise-induced myocardial ischemia (decreased blood flow to the heart) or left ventricular dysfunction.

Waiting period before certification: At least 2 months after an acute MI.

Maximum certification period: 1 year

Certification recommendations:

 Certify if the driver:
- Has no symptoms,

- Tolerates medications,

- Has a satisfactory exercise tolerance test (ETT),

- Has a resting left ventricular ejection fraction (LVEF, the amount of blood expelled when the heart contracts) greater than or equal to 40%, and

- Has no electrocardiogram ischemic changes.

NOTE: For an initial certification following an MI, an in-hospital post-MI echocardiogram showing an LVEF greater than or equal to 40% is sufficient.

✗ Do not certify if the driver has:
- Chest pain at rest, or a change in chest-pain patterns within 3 months of examination,
- Ischemic (blood supply) changes on an electrocardiogram (ECG) taken at rest, or
- Intolerance to cardiovascular therapy.

Monitoring/testing: The driver should get clearance from a cardiovascular specialist who understands the demands of commercial driving, and have a biennial ETT. Drivers in a rehabilitation program can receive comprehensive secondary prevention therapy.

Follow-up: Annual medical exams.

2. Angina Pectoris

Angina pectoris (chest pain) is at the lower end of the spectrum for risk among individuals with coronary heart disease (CHD). The presence of this condition usually implies that at least one coronary artery has significant narrowing.

When evaluating a driver with angina, the examiner will need to distinguish between stable and unstable angina. Unstable angina could lead to a disqualifying cardiovascular episode.

Stable angina	Unstable angina
May be triggered by a predictable pattern, including: • Exertion, • Emotion, • Extremes in weather, and/or • Sexual activity.	Has an unpredictable course characterized by: • Pain occurring at rest, • Changes in pattern (i.e., increased frequency and longer duration), and • Decreased response to medication.

Waiting period before certification, for stable angina: At least 3 months with no angina at rest or change in angina pattern.

Maximum certification period: 1 year

Certification recommendations:

 Certify if the driver:
  • Has stable angina with no symptoms,

  • Tolerates medications, and

  • Has a satisfactory exercise tolerance test (ETT).

✗ Do not certify if the driver has had unstable angina within 3 months of examination.

Monitoring/testing: The driver should get an evaluation from a cardiovascular specialist who understands the demands of commercial driving, and an ETT every 2 years. If an ETT is inconclusive, an imaging stress test may be needed.

Follow-up: Annual medical exams.

3. CHD "Risk-Equivalent" Conditions

The presence of one or more of these medical conditions may be insufficient to disqualify a driver. However, the presence of these conditions can cause the driver to be at as great a risk of sudden death or incapacitation as a driver with known coronary heart disease (CHD).

CHD risk-equivalent conditions include:

• The presence of diabetes mellitus;

• The presence of peripheral vascular disease;

• A Framingham risk score predicting a 20% CHD event risk over the next 10 years (see Framingham Heart Study, Risk Score Profiles); or

• Being over 45 years of age with multiple risk factors for CHD.

Waiting period before certification: As needed until the cause is confirmed and treatment is adequate, effective, safe, and stable.

Maximum certification: 1 year

Certification recommendations:

 Certify if the nature and severity of the driver's medical condition does not endanger the health and safety of the driver and the public.

NOTE: The decision not to medically certify a driver should not depend solely on the detection of multiple risk factors.

Monitoring/testing: The driver should have ongoing treating-provider follow-up, and aggressive, comprehensive risk-factor management.

Follow-up: Annual medical exams.

4. Coronary Artery Bypass Grafting Surgery

Coronary artery bypass grafting (CABG) surgery is frequently the preferred choice of therapy for individuals with multi-vessel coronary heart disease, narrowing of the proximal left main coronary artery, and extensive atherosclerosis (hardening of the arteries) in the presence of left ventricular dysfunction or debilitating chest pain.

Following CABG surgery, individuals are at less risk of sudden death than those who are treated medically. Most drivers who undergo CABG surgery are able to return to work. A longer waiting period is recommended to allow for healing of the sternal incision. The sternum should be completely healed before certifying a driver.

A significant risk associated with CABG surgery is the high long-term reocclusion (blockage) rate of the bypass graft.

STANDARDS

Waiting period before certification: At least 3 months after surgery, regardless of the type of CABG surgery performed.

Maximum certification period: 1 year

Certification recommendations:

 Certify if the driver:
  • Has no symptoms;

  • Tolerates cardiovascular medications with no symptoms brought about by the act of standing up;

  • Has a left ventricular ejection fraction (LVEF, the amount of blood expelled when the heart contracts) greater than or equal to 40%;

  • Is examined and approved by a cardiologist for medical fitness to drive; and

  • Has a healed sternum.

✗ Do not certify if any of the above conditions are not met.

Monitoring/testing: Because of the risk of re-blockage over time, 5 years post-CABG surgery, the driver should obtain:

• An annual exercise tolerance test, and

• An imaging stress test, if indicated.

Follow-up: Annual medical exams.

5. Heart Failure

The prognosis for heart failure depends on the underlying disease; however, the driving risks for heart failure do not. Sudden death is responsible for 10% to 30% of all deaths in individuals with severe symptoms. Even in mildly symptomatic individuals, sudden death accounts for the majority of deaths.

- Coronary heart disease (CHD) is the major cause of systolic dysfunction.

- Hypertension is the cause or associated factor in the development of heart failure among individuals with a non-ischemic cause.

- A weakened, enlarged heart due to an unknown cause (idiopathic dilated cardiomyopathy) is the most frequent diagnosis of individuals who have systolic dysfunction and no evidence of significant underlying coronary artery disease.

NOTE: "Congestive heart failure" is the terminology used in the *Cardiovascular Advisory Panel Guidelines for the Medical Examination of Commercial Motor Vehicle Drivers.*

Waiting period before certification: The driver should not be certified until the cause is confirmed and treatment has been shown to be adequate, effective, safe, and stable.

Maximum certification period: 1 year

Certification recommendations:

 Certify if the driver:
- Has no symptoms upon examination;

- Tolerates medication;

- Has exercise tolerance test results greater than 6 METs (metabolic equivalents); and

- Has a left ventricular ejection fraction (LVEF, the amount of blood expelled when the heart contracts) greater than or equal to 40%.

✗ Do not certify if the driver:
- Has symptomatic heart failure regardless of systolic function,

173

- Is asymptomatic with an LVEF less than or equal to 50% and has ventricular arrhythmias (sustained or nonsustained ventricular tachycardia or symptomatic palpitations), or

- Is asymptomatic and has an LVEF less than 40%.

Monitoring/testing: The driver should obtain annual evaluation and clearance from a cardiovascular specialist who understands the demands of commercial driving, including echocardiography and holter monitoring.

Follow-up: Annual medical exams.

6. Percutaneous Coronary Intervention

The *Cardiovascular Advisory Panel Guidelines for the Medical Examination of Commercial Motor Vehicle Drivers* recommendations for percutaneous coronary intervention (PCI) encompass angioplasty and other catheter-based techniques aimed at relieving coronary obstructions.

In the setting of an uncomplicated, elective procedure to treat stable angina (chest pain), the post-procedure waiting period is 1 week. The waiting period allows for a small threat caused by acute complications at the vascular access site. Drivers undergoing PCI in the setting of an acute myocardial infarction or unstable angina should be restricted from driving duties for the longer waiting period recommended for these conditions.

Waiting period before certification: At least 1 week after PCI

Maximum certification period: Initially, certification should be for up to 6 months. Recertification can be for up to 1 year if exercise tolerance test (ETT) results are satisfactory.

Certification recommendations:

 Certify if the driver:
- Shows no symptoms at examination,
- Tolerates medications, and
- Has no injury to the vascular access site.

✗ Do not certify if the driver has:
- Incomplete healing or complication at the vascular access site,
- Chest pains at rest, or
- Ischemic electrocardiogram (ECG) changes.

Monitoring/testing: Following initial certification, the driver should have an ETT 3 to 6 months after the PCI and should bring the results to a 6-month follow-up exam. The driver should get clearance from a cardiovascular specialist who understands the demands of commercial driving, and an ETT every 2 years. If an ETT is inconclusive, an imaging stress test may be necessary.

Follow-up: Annual medical exams. After PCI, typical angina symptoms should prompt evaluation with a stress imaging study or repeat angiography.

Congenital Heart Disease

Heart failure and sudden death are the major causes of death among individuals with congenital (dating from birth) heart disease. Due to the complexity of these problems, it is recommended that the driver have regular, ongoing follow-up by a cardiologist knowledgeable in adult congenital heart disease.

175

VI. Qualification Standards

Certification Recommendations:

A driver with congenital heart disease must meet the qualification standards. The medical examiner's decision to certify should be based on:

- Anatomic diagnosis,
- Severity of the congenital defect,
- Results of treatment,
- Present fitness status, and
- Risk of sudden death or incapacitation.

NOTE: *The Cardiovascular Advisory Panel Guidelines for the Medical Examination of Commercial Motor Vehicle Drivers* (see "Online Resources" in Chapter 9) discusses multiple congenital heart diseases, many of which are self-limiting. Advances in surgical and medical management are expected to result in an increased number of individuals with congenital heart disease seeking driver certification. The "Ebstein anomaly" is included below because it is a condition an examiner is likely to encounter in the clinical setting.

Ebstein Anomaly

The Ebstein anomaly is a congenital heart defect causing downward displacement of the tricuspid valve. The medical history of a patient with Ebstein anomaly depends on its severity. Adults with a mild form of Ebstein anomaly may show no symptoms throughout their lives.

Waiting period before certification: As needed until the cause is confirmed and treatment is adequate, effective, safe, and stable.

Maximum certification: 1 year

Certification recommendations:

 <u>Certify</u> if the driver:
- Is not showing symptoms,
- Has a mild tricuspid anomaly,
- Has mild cardiac enlargement, or
- Has mild right ventricular dysfunction.

✗ <u>Do not certify</u> if the driver has a(n):
- Moderate or severe anomaly,
- Intracardiac lesion,
- Shunt,
- Symptomatic arrhythmia, or
- Accessory conduction pathway.

Monitoring/testing: Annual cardiovascular re-evaluation should include echocardiography and evaluation by a cardiologist knowledgeable in adult congenital heart disease and who understands the demands of commercial driving.

Follow-up: Annual medical exams.

Heart Transplantation

Although the number of heart transplant recipients is relatively small, some recipients may wish to be commercial motor vehicle drivers. The major medical concerns for certification of a heart recipient are transplant rejection and post-transplant atherosclerosis.

Waiting period before certification: At least 1 year after transplant

Maximum certification period: 6 months

Certification recommendations:

 Certify if the driver:
- Is not showing symptoms,
- Tolerates medications,
- Has clearance from a cardiovascular specialist who understands the demands of commercial driving,
- Has no signs of transplant rejection, and
- Meets all other qualification requirements.

Monitoring/testing: Monitoring the driver with a heart transplant should include re-evaluation and recertification every 6 months by a cardiovascular specialist who:

- Is an expert in the fields of cardiology and transplant medicine;
- Understands the demands of commercial driving; and
- Evaluates the possibility of atherosclerosis, the status of the transplant, and the general health of the driver.

Follow-up: Medical exams every 6 months

Myocardial Disease

Myocardial diseases (diseases of the heart wall) are often progressive and require long-term follow-up. Even so, improved diagnostic testing and treatment can increase the number of drivers with myocardial disease who seek certification. The following myocardial diseases are disqualifying.

Hypertrophic Cardiomyopathy

Hypertrophic cardiomyopathy (a thickening of the heart wall) is a complex heart disease with diverse characteristics. Some individuals experience a benign and stable clinical course, while in others the disease is characterized by progressive symptoms. For some individuals, sudden death is the first definitive manifestation of the disease.

Restrictive Cardiomyopathy

Restrictive cardiomyopathy is a condition in which the walls of the lower chambers of the heart lose their flexibility. The Mayo Clinic studied restrictive cardiomyopathy between 1979 and 1996 and found a five-year survival rate of only 64%, compared with an expected survival rate of 85%.

Waiting period before certification: If the driver has an enlarged heart or the examiner suspects restrictive cardiomyopathy, the driver should not be certified until being evaluated by a cardiovascular specialist who understands the demands of commercial driving, to confirm or rule out a diagnosis of hypertrophic cardiomyopathy or restrictive cardiomyopathy.

Certification recommendations:

✗ <u>Do not certify</u> if the driver is diagnosed with hypertrophic cardiomyopathy or restrictive cardiomyopathy.

Syncope

Syncope (fainting) is a symptom – not a medical condition – that can present an immediate threat to public safety by causing a driver to lose control of the vehicle.

As an example, a fainting spell brought about by an irregular heartbeat while driving puts the driver and the traveling public in serious jeopardy. Medications are available that are effective in managing ventricular arrhythmias and, although they are designed to prevent occurrences, they are not "fail-safe" and if an arrhythmia recurs, syncope may follow.

Recurrent, unexplained syncope and syncope from cardiac causes may signify an increased future risk for sudden death.

The medical examiner needs to make sure that:

- Diagnosis distinguishes between pre-syncope (i.e., dizziness, lightheadedness) and true syncope (i.e., loss of consciousness);

- The driver's medications do not predispose the driver to rapid declines in blood pressure, syncope, fatigue, or electrolyte shifts and imbalances;

- Cardiac-based syncope is differentiated from other causes of syncope (conduction system diseases that cause syncope must be treated before the driver is considered for certification); and

- Other forms of syncope, such as neurological-based conditions (e.g., migraine headache, seizures) are adequately evaluated.

For specific recommendations for hypersensitive carotid sinus with syncope or neurocardiogenic syncope, refer to the *Cardiovascular Advisory Panel Guidelines for the Medical Examination of Commercial Motor Vehicle Drivers* (see "Online Resources" in Chapter 9).

Waiting period before certification: As needed until the cause is confirmed and treatment is adequate, effective, safe, and stable. If applicable, refer to the pacemaker guidelines.

Maximum certification period: 1 year

Certification recommendations:

 Certify if the driver:
- Has been treated for the disease that was causing syncope;
- Is not showing symptoms;
- Tolerates medications;
- Is at low risk for syncope/near syncope; and
- Has clearance from an appropriate specialist (e.g., cardiologist, neurologist) who understands the demands of commercial driving.

✗ Do not certify if the driver:
- Experiences syncope as a consequence of the disease process, regardless of the underlying condition; or
- Is at high risk for syncope/near syncope, regardless of the underlying heart disease and/or treatment.

Monitoring/testing: The driver should:
- Comply with medication and/or treatment guidelines, when appropriate; and
- Have annual evaluation by a cardiovascular specialist who understands the demands of commercial driving (refer to diagnosis-specific recommendations).

Follow-up: Annual medical exams.

STANDARDS

181

Valvular Heart Diseases

Murmurs – unusual swishing sounds in the heart – are a common sign of valve problems; however, the presence of a murmur may be associated with other cardiovascular conditions. The medical examiner must distinguish between functional murmurs and pathological murmurs that are medically disqualifying.

Classification of Murmurs:

The intensity of murmurs is classified on a scale of I to VI, from the least pronounced murmur to the loudest. Classification is rated as follows:

Grade	Description
I	Must strain to hear a murmur.
II	Can hear a faint murmur without straining.
III	Can easily hear a moderately loud murmur.
IV	Can easily hear a moderately loud murmur that has a thrill.
V	Can hear the murmur when only part of the stethoscope is in contact with the skin.
VI	Can hear the murmur with the stethoscope close to the skin; it does not have to be in contact with the skin to detect the murmur.

Murmurs that are (a) systolic and grade I or II or (b) mid-systolic are usually harmless if the driver has no signs or symptoms of heart disease.

Additional evaluation is recommended when murmurs are:

- Systolic, grade I or II, and the driver has signs or symptoms of heart disease;

- Systolic and grade III or higher;

- Holosystolic or late systolic; or

- Diastolic or continuous.

Exceptions are common with the higher-grade murmurs. When the examiner is in doubt about the severity of a heart murmur, he/she may seek additional evaluation.

1. Aortic Regurgitation

Severity: Mild or Moderate

Maximum certification period: 1 year

Certification recommendations:

✓ Certify if the driver is not showing symptoms.

✗ Do not certify if the driver has:
  • Symptoms,
  • Moderate aortic regurgitation with abnormal left ventricle (LV) function, or
  • More than mild LV enlargement.

Monitoring/testing: Echocardiography every 2 to 3 years

Follow-up: Annual medical exams.

Severity: Severe

Waiting period before certification: 3 months after aortic valve repair

Maximum certification: 6 months if not surgically repaired, 1 year if repaired

STANDARDS

183

Certification recommendations:

 Certify if the driver has:
- No symptoms,
- Normal left ventricle (LV) function,
- LV end-diastolic dimension (LVEDD) less than or equal to 60 mm, and
- LV end-systolic dimension (LVESD) less than or equal to 50 mm.

✕ Do not certify if the driver:
- Shows symptoms,
- Is unable to achieve workload greater than 6 METS on the Bruce protocol,
- Has reduced left ventricular ejection fraction less than 50%,
- Has LVEDD greater than 70 mm, or
- Has LVESD greater than 55 mm.

Monitoring/testing: Echocardiography every 4 to 12 months

Follow-up: Semi-annual medical exams, or annual if surgically repaired.

2. Aortic Stenosis

Waiting period before certification: 3 months after surgery

Maximum certification period: 1 year

Certification recommendations:

 Certify if the condition is:
- *Mild* and the driver has no symptoms;
- *Moderate* with no symptoms and the driver has no disqualifying findings and/or conditions; or
- *Severe* but has been surgically repaired and meets all surgical guidelines for aortic valve repair.

✗ Do not certify if the condition is:
- *Moderate* and the driver has one or more of the following: angina, heart failure, atrial fibrillation, left ventricular dysfunction with ejection fraction less than 50%, or thromboembolism; or
- *Severe*.

Monitoring/testing: Echocardiography every 5 years if mild or every 1 to 2 years if moderate.

Follow-up: Annual medical exams

3. Aortic Valve Repair

Waiting period before certification: 3 months after repair

Maximum certification period: 1 year

Certification recommendations:

 Certify if the driver meets asymptomatic aortic stenosis or aortic regurgitation qualification requirements (as outlined above) and has clearance

185

from a cardiovascular specialist who understands the demands of commercial driving.

✗ <u>Do not certify</u> if the driver has complications from the blocking of a blood vessel by a blood clot dislodged from its site of origin (thromboembolism).

Monitoring/testing: Two-dimensional echocardiography with Doppler prior to discharge; additional monitoring and testing based on aortic regurgitation severity.

Follow-up: Annual medical exams

4. Mitral Regurgitation

Waiting period before certification: 3 months after surgery

Maximum certification period: 1 year

Certification recommendations:

 <u>Certify</u> if the driver has:
  - Mild or moderate condition with no symptoms, normal left ventricular (LV) size and function, and normal pulmonary artery pressure;

  - Severe condition with no symptoms; or

  - Surgical mitral valve repair with no symptoms, and has clearance from a cardiovascular specialist who understands the demands of commercial driving.

✗ <u>Do not certify</u> if the driver has symptoms, less than 6 METs on the the Bruce protocol, ruptured chordae or flail leaflet, atrial fibrillation, LV dysfunction, thromboembolism, or pulmonary hypertension.

Monitoring/testing:

- Moderate condition: Annual echocardiography

- Severe condition: Exercise tolerance test and echocardiography every 6 to 12 months.

Follow-up: Annual medical exams

5. Mitral Stenosis

Waiting period before certification: 4 weeks after percutaneous balloon mitral valvotomy; 3 months after surgical commissurotomy.

Maximum certification period: 1 year

Certification recommendations:

 Certify if the driver has:
- Mild or moderate condition with no symptoms; or
- Severe condition and clearance from a cardio-vascular specialist who understands the demands of commercial driving following percutaneous balloon mitral valvotomy or surgical commissurotomy.

✕ Do not certify if the condition is severe and untreated.

Monitoring/testing: At least annual evaluation by a cardiovascular specialist, including chest X-ray, electrocardiogram, and two-dimensional echocardiography with Doppler or other mitral stenosis severity assessment.

Follow-up: Annual medical exams

6. Mitral Valve Prolapse

Waiting period before certification: As needed until the cause is confirmed and treatment is adequate, effective, safe, and stable.

187

VI. Qualification Standards

Maximum certification period: 1 year

Certification recommendations:

✓ Certify if the nature and severity of the condition does not endanger the health and safety of the driver and the public.

✗ Do not certify if the driver has symptoms or reduced effort tolerance due to mitral valve prolapse or mitral regurgitation; ruptured chordae or flail leaflet; systemic emboli; atrial fibrillation; syncope or documented ventricular tachycardia; or severe mitral regurgitation or LV dysfunction.

Monitoring/testing: Exercise tolerance testing may be helpful to assess symptoms. Drivers with definite mitral regurgitation (even if mild), or markedly thickened leaflets, should have annual echocardiography and clearance from a cardiovascular specialist who understands the demands of commercial driving.

Follow-up: Annual medical exams

7. Mitral Valve Repair for Mitral Regurgitation

Waiting period before certification: 3 months after repair

Maximum certification period: 1 year

Certification recommendations:

✓ Certify if the driver does not have symptoms and meets the underlying mild, moderate, or severe mitral regurgitation recommendations (see above). The driver should also have clearance from a cardiovascular specialist who understands the demands of commercial driving.

✗ Do not certify if the driver has thromboembolic complications, atrial fibrillation, or pulmonary hypertension.

Monitoring/testing: Additional tests and/or consultation as needed.

Follow-up: Annual medical exams

8. Prosthetic Valves

Waiting period before certification: 3 months after valve replacement

Maximum certification period: 1 year

Certification recommendations:

✓ Certify if the driver has no symptoms and has clearance from a cardiovascular specialist who understands the demands of commercial driving.

✗ Do not certify if the driver has persistent symptoms, LV dysfunction (ejection fraction less than 40%), thromboembolic complications, atrial fibrillation, pulmonary hypertension, or inadequate anticoagulation based on monthly International Normalized Ratio (INR) checks (INR is a measure of the ability of blood to clot).

Monitoring/testing: If treatment includes anticoagulant therapy, the driver should meet INR monitoring guidelines. Echocardiography is appropriate if there are concerns about prosthetic valve dysfunction, perivalvular leaks, new murmurs, or LV function. Exercise tolerance testing may be required to assess work capacity.

Follow-up: Annual medical exams

9. Pulmonary Valve Stenosis

Waiting period before certification: 1 month after balloon valvuloplasty, 3 months after surgical valvotomy.

Maximum certification period: 1 year

Certification recommendations:

✓ Certify if the driver has a mild or moderate condition or if the condition was corrected by surgical valvotomy or balloon valvuloplasty.

✗ Do not certify if the driver has:

- Symptoms of difficulty breathing, palpitations, or fainting;

- Pulmonary valve peak gradient greater than 50 mm Hg in the presence of a normal cardiac output;

- Right ventricular pressure greater than 50% systemic pressure;

- More than mild right ventricular hypertrophy noted by echocardiography;

- More than mild right ventricular dysfunction noted by echocardiography;

- More than moderate pulmonary valve regurgitation noted by echocardiography; or

- Main pulmonary artery diameter more than 5 cm noted by echocardiography or other imaging method.

Monitoring/testing: Driver should have annual cardiology evaluations by a cardiovascular specialist who is knowledgeable in adult congenital heart disease and who understands the demands of commercial driving.

Follow-up: Annual medical exams

Respiratory

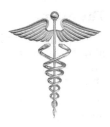

The standard: §391.41(b)(5)

A person is physically qualified to drive a commercial motor vehicle (CMV) if that person has no established medical history or clinical diagnosis of a respiratory dysfunction likely to interfere with his/her ability to control and drive a CMV safely.

Public safety considerations:

The commercial driver spends more time driving than the average individual. Driving is a repetitive and monotonous activity that demands the driver be alert at all times. Symptoms of respiratory dysfunction or disease can be debilitating and can interfere with the ability to remain attentive to driving conditions and to perform heavy exertion. Even the slightest impairment in respiratory function under emergency conditions (when greater oxygen supply may be necessary for performance) can be harmful to safe driving.

There are many primary and secondary respiratory conditions that interfere with oxygen exchange and may result in gradual or sudden incapacitation, such as:

- Asthma

- Carcinoma

- Chronic bronchitis

- Emphysema

- Obstructive sleep apnea

- Tuberculosis

In addition, medications used to treat respiratory conditions, both prescription and those available without a prescription, may cause cognitive difficulties, compound the risk for excessive daytime sleepiness, or cause other forms of incapacitation.

191

The exam:

The examiner will discuss and document information about any respiratory-related symptoms the driver may have, such as shortness of breath, asthma, sleepiness, or loud snoring.

Based on the findings of the physical exam, the medical examiner may request a detailed pulmonary function evaluation or consultation with a pulmonologist.

The examiner must document any discussion with the driver about history, medication, and abnormal findings concerning the respiratory system.

Allergies and Asthma-Related Diseases

Allergies are common in the general population; however, mild symptoms don't interfere with safe driving. Severe symptoms can affect lung function, cause breathing difficulty, low blood oxygen, cognitive dysfunction, anxiety, panic, or diminished levels of consciousness.

A driver at risk for sudden onset of symptoms that interfere with safe driving should have documentation of successful preventive measures and/or treatment undertaken without adverse effects before being certified as medically fit for duty.

1. Allergic Rhinitis

Allergic rhinitis, which involves inflammation of the nasal portion of the upper respiratory tract, should rarely render the driver medically unqualified for commercial driving. The symptoms should be treated with non-sedating antihistamines or with local steroid sprays that do not interfere with driving ability.

Maximum certification: 2 years

Certification recommendations:

 Certify if:
- The cause is confirmed;
- Treatment is adequate, effective, safe, and stable; and
- The examiner believes the nature and severity of the condition does not endanger the health and safety of the driver and the public.

✗ Do not certify if the driver has complications and/or treatment that impairs function, including:
- Severe conjunctivitis affecting vision,
- Inability to keep eyes open,
- Sensitivity to light,
- Uncontrollable sneezing fits,
- Sinusitis with severe headaches, or
- Medications that cause sedation or other side effects that interfere with safe driving.

Monitoring/testing: Additional tests and/or consultation may be needed.

Follow-up: Follow-up depends on the clinical course of the condition and recommendation of the treating healthcare provider.

2. Allergy-Related Life-Threatening Conditions

These conditions encompass systemic anaphylaxis and acute upper airway obstruction induced by allergens, genetic deficiencies, or unknown mechanisms, including:

- Stinging insect allergy that may result in acute anaphylaxis following a sting. Preventive measures include carrying an epinephrine injection device in the truck cab and evaluating the driver for immunotherapy.

- Hereditary or acquired angioedema (swelling below the skin surface) that may result in an acute, life-threatening airway obstruction or severe abdominal pain requiring urgent medical attention. Prevention and control can and should be accomplished with appropriate medication.

- Acute recurrent episodes of idiopathic anaphylaxis or angioedema that may occur unpredictably in some individuals and lead to sudden onset of severe breathing difficulty, visual disturbance, loss of consciousness, or collapse. Similar episodes occur due to known allergens, including medications, which ordinarily can be avoided.

Waiting period before certification: Drivers with a history of an allergy-related life-threatening condition must have undertaken successful preventive measures and/or treatment without adverse effects before the driver can be considered medically qualified.

Maximum certification: 2 years

Certification recommendations:

✔ Certify if the nature and severity of the condition and the prevention and treatment regimen do not endanger the health and safety of the driver and the public.

✘ Do not certify if the driver with a history of an allergy-related life-threatening condition does not have an effective treatment regimen or successful preventive measures.

Monitoring/testing: The examiner may order additional tests and/or consultation as necessary.

Follow-up: Follow-up depends on the clinical course of the condition and recommendations of the treating healthcare provider.

3. Asthma

Individuals with asthma generally exhibit reversible airway obstruction that can be treated effectively with medication such as bronchodilators and corticosteroids; however, asthma ranges in severity from essentially no symptoms to potentially fatal. In some drivers, complications of asthma and/or side effects of therapy may interfere with safe driving.

Waiting period before certification: As needed until the cause is confirmed and treatment is adequate, effective, safe, and stable.

Maximum certification: 2 years

Certification recommendations:

✕ Do not certify if the driver exhibits either:
  - Continual, uncontrolled, symptomatic asthma; OR
  - Significant impairment of pulmonary function (forced expiratory volume in the first second of expiration (FEV1) less than 65%) and significant hypoxemia (partial pressure of arterial oxygen (PaO2) less than 65 mm Hg).

Monitoring/testing: The examiner may order additional tests and/or consultation as necessary.

Follow-up: Follow-up depends on the course of the condition and recommendations of the treating healthcare provider.

4. Hypersensitivity Pneumonitis

Hypersensitivity pneumonitis is an immune-mediated granulomatous interstitial pneumonitis (inflammation of the lungs) that may present itself as an acute recurrent, sub-acute, or chronic illness variously manifested by shortness of breath, cough, and fever. The condition may not prevent an individual from qualifying for commercial driving; however, a driver with this condition requires medical care to alleviate symptoms.

➤ **The driver should avoid exposure to whatever causes the symptoms (e.g., transporting the agent) because severe respiratory impairment could occur with repeated exposure.**

Waiting period before certification: As needed until the cause is confirmed and treatment is adequate, effective, safe, and stable.

Maximum certification: 2 years

Certification recommendations:

✗ Do not certify if the nature and severity of the driver's medical condition endangers the health and safety of the driver and the public.

Monitoring/testing: A chest X-ray may be necessary to reveal lung disease.

Follow-up: Biennial medical exams (every 2 years)

Chronic Obstructive Pulmonary Disease

Chronic obstructive pulmonary disease (COPD) is not a single disease, but a group of medical conditions characterized by a chronic reduction in the amount of air that can be breathed out, most often caused by chronic bronchitis or emphysema.

Most drivers with COPD have a combination of chronic bronchitis and emphysema. COPD develops slowly with few initial symptoms. The driver may have substantial reduction in lung function prior to developing breathing difficulties on exertion. The cardinal symptoms are:

• Chronic cough,

• Sputum production, and/or

• Breathing difficulties with exertion.

As the disease progresses, these symptoms can become incapacitating. In the majority of cases, cigarette smoking is a primary causal factor.

Waiting period before certification: As needed until the cause is confirmed and treatment is adequate, effective, safe, and stable.

Maximum certification: 2 years

Certification recommendations:

- ✓ Certify if the condition is stable and does not endanger driver or public health or safety.

- ✗ Do not certify if the driver has hypoxemia (low blood oxygen) at rest, chronic respiratory failure, or a history of continuing cough with cough syncope (fainting).

Monitoring/testing: Obvious difficulty breathing in a resting position indicates the need for additional pulmonary function tests. If the forced expiratory volume in the first second of expiration (FEV1) is less than 65% of what would be expected, arterial blood gas measurements should be evaluated.

NOTE: Smokers have a high incidence of COPD, yet individuals may have a significant reduction in lung function without symptoms. The FMCSA recommends that spirometry should be performed in all smokers over the age of 35 years, to test their lung function.

Follow-up: Follow-up depends on the clinical course of the condition and recommendations of the treating healthcare provider.

Pulmonary Function Tests

Lung disorders are associated with physiological impairment, so pulmonary function testing (PFT) may be necessary. Signs pointing to the need for PFT include:

- A history of any specific lung disease;

- Symptoms of shortness of breath, cough, chest tightness, or wheezing; or

- Cigarette smoking in drivers 35 years of age or older.

Spirometry (Airflow Measurement)

When the above indicators are present, the examiner should measure the driver's lung function, including "forced expiratory volume in the first second of expiration" (FEV1), "forced vital capacity" (FVC), and the FEV1/FVC ratio. No further testing is necessary if the lung function is normal and no other abnormality is suspected. Abnormal lung function should be further evaluated.

Screening Pulse Oximetry And/Or Arterial Blood Gas (ABG) Analysis

These tests are appropriate when:

- The condition causes airway obstruction and pulmonary function test results are:

    - FEV1 is less than 65% of the predicted value.

    - The FEV1/FVC ratio is less than 65%.

- Restrictive impairment is present and FVC is less than 60%.

Screening Pulse Oximetry

If oximetry (blood-oxygen saturation) is less than 92% (oximetry equals 70), the driver must have an ABG analysis.

Arterial Blood Gas (ABG) Analysis

The driver should not be certified when ABG measurements reveal:

- Partial pressure of arterial oxygen (PaO2) of less than:

  - 65 mm Hg at altitudes below 5,000 feet, or

  - 60 mm Hg at altitudes above 5,000 feet.

- Partial pressure of arterial carbon dioxide (PaCO2) greater than 45 mm Hg at any altitude.

Chronic Sleep Disorders

Approximately 70% of the cases of excessive daytime sleepiness (EDS) are caused by narcolepsy and obstructive sleep apnea (OSA).

Treatments for OSA include surgery and continuous positive airway pressure (CPAP). A successfully treated driver may be considered for certification following the recommended waiting period. Drivers with suspected or untreated sleep apnea should not be certified until the cause is confirmed and treatment is stable, safe, adequate, and effective.

> **NOTE:** Refer to the Reference area for an FMCSA bulletin on obstructive sleep apnea.

EDS may also be a symptom of another underlying condition, such as:

- Neurological disease,

- Depression,

- Alcohol or other drug use, or

- Prescription and/or over-the-counter medication use.

Waiting period before certification: At least 1 month after starting CPAP; at least 3 months symptom free after surgical treatment.

Maximum certification: 1 year

Certification recommendations:

 Certify if the driver has:
- Successful non-surgical therapy with "multiple sleep-latency testing" values (i.e., the time it takes to fall asleep) within the normal range and resolution of apneas confirmed by repeated sleep studies during treatment;
- Continuous successful non-surgical therapy for 1 month;
- Compliance with continuing non-surgical therapy; and/or
- Resolution of symptoms following completion of the post-surgical waiting period.

✕ Do not certify if the driver has:
- Hypoxemia (low blood oxygen) at rest; or
- A diagnosis of untreated symptomatic OSA, narcolepsy, primary (idiopathic) alveolar hypoventilation syndrome, idiopathic central nervous system hypersomnolence, or restless leg syndrome associated with EDS.

Monitoring/testing: A driver who is being treated for sleep apnea should remain symptom free and agree to continue uninterrupted therapy and undergo yearly objective testing (e.g., "multiple sleep-latency" testing or "maintenance of wakefulness" testing).

Follow-up: Follow-up depends on the clinical course of the condition and recommendations of the treating healthcare provider, not to exceed 1 year.

Sleep Disorder Tests

1. Objective tests for sleep disorders

When indicated, objective sleep tests may be required to determine the presence of a sleep disorder. These tests include polysomnography in a controlled sleep laboratory and napping tests ("maintenance of wakefulness" test and "multiple sleep-latency test").

Definitions:

- Apnea — airflow ceases for more than 10 seconds.

- Hypopnea — airflow decreases for more than 10 seconds.

Severity (apnea-hypopnea index):

- Mild – 5 or more episodes per hour.

- Moderate – 15 or more episodes per hour.

- Severe – 30 or more episodes per hour.

More than 30 episodes per hour of sleep is considered a diagnosis of obstructive sleep apnea.

2. Self-reported sleepiness surveys

Simple sleepiness surveys may be useful for obtaining a driver's self-assessment of his/her degree of sleepiness. Examples of sleepiness surveys include:

- The Epworth sleepiness scale,

- The Stanford sleepiness scale, and

- The "functional outcomes of sleep" questionnaire.

NOTE: Self-reported sleepiness does NOT always correlate with objective testing (polysomnography). The driver may not perceive sleepiness as excessive or may be hesitant to disclose sleepiness.

For more information, see: *Tech Brief: A Study of Prevalence of Sleep Apnea Among Commercial Truck Drivers* (see "Online Resources" in Chapter 9).

Infectious Respiratory Diseases

Although the conditions in this category are of varying cause and severity, if properly treated most have no long-term implications for driving ability. However, during acute infection, the symptoms are debilitating and can interfere with the ability to remain attentive to driving conditions and to perform heavy exertion. In addition, medications used to treat respiratory-tract congestion can cause drowsiness and loss of attention. The conditions include the common cold, influenza, acute bronchitis, pneumonia, and tuberculosis.

1. Acute Infectious Diseases

For illnesses such as the common cold, influenza, and acute bronchitis, the driver should:

- Be relieved from duty until proper treatment for the illness has been completed;

- Abstain from driving a vehicle for at least 12 hours after taking sedating medications; and

- Avoid operating a vehicle during the time that the disease is contagious.

Many of these conditions are of short duration and proper treatment for the illness must be completed before the driver returns to work.

Waiting period before certification: No recommended time frame

Maximum certification: 2 years

Certification recommendations:

✗ <u>Do not certify</u> if the nature and severity of the driver's medical condition endangers the health and safety of the driver and the public.

Monitoring/testing: Medications used to treat respiratory tract congestion, such as prescriptions and/or over-the-counter antihistamines or narcotic antitussives, can cause drowsiness and loss of attention. The driver should be educated to refrain from operating a vehicle for at least 12 hours after taking a medication with sedating side effects.

Follow-up: At least biennial medical exams (every 2 years)

2. Atypical Tuberculosis

Atypical tuberculosis (TB) covers the same broad spectrum of symptoms and disability as TB. Many individuals are "colonized" but not infected with atypical organisms, usually *Mycobacterium avium* and *Mycobacterium intracellulare*. The broad group of atypical Mycobacteria are considered noninfectious and noncontagious. The major issue to be determined is the amount of disease the patient has and the extent of the symptoms. Many cases of Mycobacteria cause very few symptoms. The X-ray findings are often migratory and are associated with cough, mild hemoptysis (coughing up of blood), and sputum production.

Atypical TB is not generally treated with medication. However, if the driver is using medication, he/she should be assessed for side effects that interfere with driving ability.

The certification issues include the amount of disease the driver has experienced and the severity of the symptoms. The potential risk is that if the disease is progressive, respiratory insufficiency may develop.

Waiting period before certification: As needed until
the cause is confirmed and treatment is adequate, effective, safe, and stable.

Maximum certification: 2 years

Certification recommendations:

✓ Certify if the disease remains relatively stable
and the driver has normal lung function and tolerates the medical regimen.

✗ Do not certify if the driver has extensive pulmonary dysfunction, weakness, fatigue, and/or adverse reaction to medical treatment.

Monitoring/testing: Pulmonary function tests should
be performed if the examiner suspects the disease has
become progressive and may cause extensive pulmonary
symptoms.

Follow-up: Follow-up depends on the clinical course of
the condition and recommendations of the treating
healthcare provider.

3. Pulmonary Tuberculosis

Although modern therapy has been extremely successful in controlling this disease, pulmonary tuberculosis
(TB) persists in some individuals while on therapy or in
individuals who are non-compliant with therapy. Advanced TB may cause respiratory insufficiency; however, risk of recurrence after adequate therapy is low.

Waiting period before certification: The driver
should not be certified until he/she is determined to be
non-contagious, the cause is confirmed, and treatment
is adequate, effective, safe, and stable.

Maximum certification: 2 years

Certification recommendations:

✓ Certify if the driver is not contagious, has completed streptomycin (antibiotic) therapy without affecting hearing and/or balance, is compliant with anti-tubercular therapy, and has no side effects that interfere with safe driving.

✗ Do not certify if the driver has:

- Advanced TB with respiratory insufficiency not meeting pulmonary function test criteria;

- Chronic TB;

- Exhibited non-compliance with anti-tubercular therapy;

- Not completed streptomycin therapy; or

- Residual eighth cranial nerve damage that affects balance and/or hearing to an extent that interferes with safe driving.

Monitoring/testing: Additional tests and/or consultation may be necessary. A positive intermediate tuberculin skin test indicates a previous TB infection. A positive purified protein derivative (PPD) skin test associated with a normal chest X-ray requires no further action. If X-ray changes are present, suggesting pulmonary TB findings, further evaluation is needed.

If the conversion occurred within the last year, active disease may develop and prophylactic therapy should take place. This circumstance would not require limiting the activities of the driver unless medication side effects and/or adverse reactions occur.

Follow-up: Follow-up depends on the clinical course of the condition and recommendations of the treating healthcare provider.

STANDARDS

Non-Infectious Respiratory Diseases

This category includes a number of diseases that cause significant long-term structural changes in the lungs and/or thorax and, therefore, interfere with the functioning of the lungs. Obvious difficulty breathing in a resting position indicates the need for additional testing.

1. Chest-Wall Deformities

Acute or chronic chest-wall deformities may affect the mechanics of breathing. Examples include kyphosis, kyphoscoliosis, pectus excavatum, ankylosing spondylitis, massive obesity, and recent thoracic/upper abdominal surgery or injury.

A driver certified with a chest-wall deformity should have near-normal airway function.

No specific medication exists for treatment. However, individuals may be particularly sensitive to the side effects of alcohol, antidepressants, and sleeping medications, even in small doses.

Waiting period before certification: As needed until the cause is confirmed and any associated treatment is adequate, effective, safe, and stable.

Maximum certification: 2 years

Certification recommendations:

   ✗ Do not certify if the driver has hypoxemia (inadequate blood oxygen) at rest, chronic respiratory failure, and/or a history of continuing cough with cough syncope (fainting).

Monitoring/testing: Obvious difficulty breathing in a resting position indicates the need for additional pulmonary function tests.

Follow-up: Follow-up depends on the clinical course of the condition and recommendations of the treating healthcare provider.

2. Chronic Obstructive Pulmonary Disease

This disease is discussed earlier in this chapter.

3. Cystic Fibrosis

Until recently, few individuals with cystic fibrosis (CF) lived into adulthood, but with modern therapy the number of survivors continues to increase. Treatment for CF may require almost continuous antibiotic therapy and daily respiratory therapy to mobilize abnormal secretions. Chronic debilitating illness may result in limited physical strength. Some individuals have a mild form of the disease that may not be diagnosed until early adulthood.

Individuals must be evaluated as to the extent of their disease and symptoms and ability to obtain therapy while working.

Waiting period before certification: As needed until treatment is adequate, effective, safe, and stable, and the driver complies with continuing medical surveillance by the appropriate specialist.

Maximum certification: 2 years; or 1 year if frequent monitoring is required.

Certification recommendations:

✗ Do not certify if the driver has:
   • Hypoxemia (inadequate blood oxygen) at rest,

   • Chronic respiratory failure,

   • A history of continuing cough with cough syncope (fainting),

   • Not met spirometry parameters, and/or

- Has an unstable condition and/or treatment regimen.

Monitoring/testing: Obvious difficulty breathing in a resting position indicates the need for additional pulmonary function tests.

Follow-up: At least annual exams, but follow-up depends on the clinical course of the condition and recommendations of the treating specialist.

4. Interstitial Lung Disease

The interstitial lung diseases (ILDs) are a varied group of diseases classified together because of common features. Occupational and environmental exposures are common causes.

A history of breathlessness while driving, walking short distances, climbing stairs, handling cargo or equipment, and entering or exiting the cab or cargo space should initiate a careful evaluation of pulmonary function for any disqualifying secondary conditions.

Although the course of ILDs is variable, progression of the disease is common and often slow to develop. Treatment side effects pose a significant potential problem because of the use of conicosteroids and cytotoxic agents.

Waiting period before certification: As needed until the cause is confirmed and treatment is adequate, effective, safe, and stable.

Maximum certification: 2 years

Certification recommendations:

✗ Do not certify if the driver has:
- Hypoxemia (inadequate blood oxygen) at rest,
- Chronic respiratory failure, or
- A history of continuing cough with cough syncope (fainting).

Monitoring/testing: Obvious difficulty breathing in a resting position indicates the need for additional pulmonary function tests.

Follow-up: Follow-up depends on the clinical course of the condition and recommendations of the treating healthcare provider.

5. Pneumothorax

Pneumothorax (air between the membranes that surround the lungs) may follow trauma to the chest or may occur spontaneously.

- **Traumatic pneumothorax** — A medical history and physical exam will provide the details of the event but may not help to ascertain recovery. Complete recovery should be confirmed by chest X-rays.

- **Spontaneous pneumothorax** — If the condition complicates an existing lung disease (such as emphysema), then the underlying lung disease will determine the chance of a recurrent pneumothorax and whether the driver can be certified.

Waiting period before certification: Complete recovery should be ensured using chest X-rays. If there is air in the pleural space and/or air in the mediastinum (pneumomediastinum) additional time away from work is indicated.

Maximum certification: 2 years

Certification recommendations:

 Certify if the driver has:

- No symptoms, with no chest pain or shortness of breath;

- No disqualifying underlying lung disease;

- Confirmed resolution of the single spontaneous pneumothorax; and/or

- Successful pleurodesis and meets acceptable pulmonary parameters.

✗ Do not certify if the driver has:

- Not met certification parameters;

- A history of two or more spontaneous pneumothoraces on one side if no successful surgical procedure has been done to prevent recurrence;

- Hypoxemia (low blood oxygen) at rest;

- Chronic respiratory failure; or

- A history of continuing cough with cough syncope (fainting).

Monitoring/testing: Chest X-rays may be necessary.

Follow-up: Follow-up depends on the clinical course of the condition and recommendations of the treating healthcare provider.

Secondary Respiratory Conditions and Underlying Disorders

The diseases or conditions in this category affect the lungs, not as a primary disease, but as a part of another disease category. Case-by-case clinical evaluation determines if the underlying condition, the symptoms, or the treatment interferes with safe driving.

1. Chronic Sleep Disorders

These disorders are discussed earlier in this chapter.

2. Cor Pulmonale

Cor pulmonale refers to enlargement of the right ventricle secondary to disorders affecting lung structure or function. In North America, the most common pulmonary cause of cor pulmonale is hypoxic pulmonary vasoconstriction in individuals with chronic obstructive pulmonary disease. The most common cause of right ventricular dilation or enlargement is pulmonary hypertension secondary to left heart disease.

The major risks are dizziness, low blood pressure, fainting, and common side effects of medications used to treat high blood pressure which may interfere with driving.

Waiting period before certification: As needed until diagnosis is confirmed and/or treatment is adequate, effective, safe, and stable.

Maximum certification: 2 years; or 1 year if frequent monitoring is required.

Certification recommendations:

X Do not certify if the driver has:
  • Breathing difficulty while at rest,

  • Dizziness,

  • Low blood pressure, and/or

  • Partial pressure of arterial oxygen (PaO_2) in arterial blood greater than 65 mm Hg.

Monitoring/testing: Additional pulmonary function tests may be needed if the driver has obvious difficulty breathing in a resting position.

Follow-up: Follow-up depends on the clinical course of the condition and recommendation of the treating healthcare provider.

---

3. Pulmonary Hypertension

Pulmonary hypertension can occur with or without cor pulmonale. Significant pulmonary hypertension is pulmonary artery pressure greater than 50% systemic systolic blood pressure from any cause.

An increased risk for incapacitation and sudden death is associated with both primary and secondary pulmonary hypertension.

Waiting period before certification: As needed until diagnosis is confirmed and/or treatment is adequate, effective, safe, and stable.

Maximum certification: 1 year

Certification recommendations:

✗ Do not certify if the driver has:
- Breathing difficulty while at rest,
- Dizziness,
- Low blood pressure, and/or
- Partial pressure of arterial oxygen (PaO2) less than 65 mm Hg.

Monitoring/testing: The examiner may order additional tests and/or consultation as necessary.

Follow-up: Follow-up depends on the clinical course of the condition and recommendations of the treating healthcare provider.

Neurological

The standard: §391.41(b)(7), (8), (9)

A person is physically qualified to drive a commercial motor vehicle (CMV) if that person:

- Has no established medical history or clinical diagnosis of rheumatic, arthritic, orthopedic, muscular, neuromuscular, or vascular disease which interferes with his/her ability to control and operate a CMV safely;

- Has no established medical history or clinical diagnosis of epilepsy or any other condition which is likely to cause loss of consciousness or any loss of ability to control a CMV; and

- Has no mental, nervous, organic, or functional disease or psychiatric disorder likely to interfere with his/her ability to drive a CMV safely.

Public safety considerations:

Drivers must remain watchful, alert, and attentive for extended periods of time in all types of traffic, road, and weather conditions. Neurological demands of driving include cognitive demands like sustained alertness, quick reactions, communication skills, and appropriate behavior, as well as physical demands like coordination.

Risks:

- **Headaches** — Most individuals have experienced the symptoms of headaches, vertigo, and dizziness. While generally harmless, these symptoms may become a problem for CMV drivers. Headache and chronic "nagging" pain may be present to such a degree that certification is inadvisable and the medication used to treat headaches may further interfere with safe driving. Disorders with incapacitating symptoms, even if periodic or in the early stages of disease, could lead to disqualification.

213

- **Vertigo and dizziness** — Multiple conditions may affect equilibrium or balance resulting in incapacitation or varying degrees of disorientation. A driver should not be certified if suffering from vertigo and/or dizziness with incapacitating symptoms that interfere with cognitive abilities, judgment, attention, concentration, and/or sensory or motor function, even if periodic or in the early stages of disease.

- **Seizures and epilepsy** — Safety is the major reason drivers with epilepsy or seizures are restricted from commercial driving. Loss of consciousness endangers the driver and the public. The physical and mental demands of commercial driving expose seizure-prone individuals to conditions that may increase the risk for seizures and may interfere with management of seizures, including:

  - Inconsistent access to medical evaluation and care for acute problems.

  - Delays in replacement of anticonvulsant medication if lost or forgotten.

The length of time an individual is seizure free and off anticonvulsant medication is considered the best predictor of future risk for seizures. Other considerations include the underlying cause of the seizure and the area of the brain affected by disease or injury.

The exam:

Many driver tasks, from load securement to turning, require physical coordination. The examiner will need to carefully consider whether a driver's neurological disease or disorder is likely to get worse, cause sudden problems while driving, and/or lead to sudden death or incapacitation.

The examiner will ask the driver about any neurological symptoms or episodes (such as seizures) and the history of injuries/illnesses, fainting/dizziness, medication use, etc.

The examiner may also observe and/or ask about the driver's appearance, hygiene, speech, coordination, alertness, and behavior.

The examiner may order additional tests and/or consultation as necessary.

STANDARDS

NOTE: Medical fitness for duty includes the ability to perform strenuous labor and requires the driver to be free of any neurological limitations that are severe enough to interfere with cognitive abilities, judgment, attention, concentration, vision, physical strength, agility, or reaction time.

Anticonvulsant Therapy

Anticonvulsant therapy is used to control or prevent seizures. Even with effective therapy there's still a risk for a seizure if the medication is inadvertently missed.

Anticonvulsants are also prescribed for other conditions that do not cause seizures, including some psychiatric disorders (for mood-stabilizing effects) and to lessen chronic pain.

Side effects may include depressed mood, cognitive deficits, decreased reflex responses, unsteadiness, and sedation.

➤ **Small doses used for chronic pain are less likely to have side effects that can interfere with safe driving than the doses used to treat other disorders.**

Waiting period before certification: As needed until the therapy is adequate, effective, safe, and stable.

Maximum certification: 2 years

Certification recommendations:

 Certify if:
- The nature and severity of the underlying condition does not interfere with safe driving, and
- The effects of medication used while driving do not endanger the safety of the driver and the public.

✕ Do not certify if the driver uses anticonvulsant medications to control or prevent seizures.

Follow-up: Annual medical exams

Episodic Neurological Conditions

Guidance on episodic neurological conditions is grouped based on the type of risk associated with the condition:

1. The types of headache, vertigo, and dizziness that can affect cognitive abilities, judgment, attention, and concentration, as well as impact sensory or motor function enough to interfere with the ability to drive safely.

2. The conditions that are known to cause or increase the risk for seizures, including epilepsy.

1. Acute Seizures Caused by Brain Injury

Individuals may have a seizure at the time of a brain injury, often depending on both the location and severity of the injury. Such individuals are often at risk for later epilepsy or unprovoked seizures. In general, the risk for subsequent unprovoked seizures is greatest in the first 2 years following the injury.

The length of time an individual is seizure free and off anticonvulsant medication is considered the best predictor of future risk for seizures. Therefore, according to medical guidelines, for the entire waiting period before being considered for certification, the driver should be both:

• Seizure-free, and

• Off anticonvulsant medication prescribed for control of seizures.

Drivers should NOT be considered for certification if they:

• Survive a *severe* head injury, because the risk for developing unprovoked seizures does not decrease significantly over time;

• Have a surgical procedure involving penetration of the outermost membrane around the brain and spinal cord (dura mater), because such drivers have a risk for subsequent epilepsy similar to that of severe head trauma; or

• Have had surgery for epilepsy.

Waiting period before certification:

If seizure free and off anticonvulsant medication following:	then wait at least:
• Mild injury without early seizures, • Stroke without risk for seizures, or • Intracerebral or subarachnoid hemorrhage without risk for seizures	1 year.
• Moderate injury without early seizures, or • Mild injury with early seizures	2 years.
• Moderate injury with early seizures, • Stroke with risk for seizures, or • Intracerebral or subarachnoid hemorrhage with risk for seizures	5 years.

Maximum certification: 1 year

Certification recommendations:

 Certify if the driver with a history of mild or moderate injury has:
- Completed the minimum waiting period;
- Normal physical exam, neurological exam including neuro-ophthalmological evaluation, and neuropsychological test; and
- Clearance from a neurologist who understands the demands of commercial driving.

✕ Do not certify if the driver has a history of a severe brain injury with or without early seizures.

Follow-up: Annual medical exams

2. Acute Seizures Caused by Systemic Illness

Seizures are the normal reaction of a properly functioning nervous system in the presence of systemic metabolic illness, and are not known to be associated with any inherent tendency to have further seizures. The risk for additional seizures is related to the likelihood of the systemic illness coming back.

Waiting period before certification: As needed until the cause is confirmed and treatment is adequate, effective, safe, and stable.

Maximum certification: 2 years

Certification recommendations:

 Certify if:
- The underlying systemic metabolic dysfunction has been corrected; and
- The driver has no disqualifying risk of recurrence of the primary condition.

Follow-up: At least biennial medical exams (every 2 years)

218

3. Childhood Febrile Seizures

Febrile seizures are brought on by a fever, and they occur in 2-5% of children in the United States before 5 years of age and seldom occur after 5 years of age. From a practical standpoint, most individuals who have experienced a febrile seizure in infancy are unaware of the event and the condition cannot be discovered through routine screening. Most of the increased risk for unprovoked seizure is found in the first 10 years of life.

Waiting period before certification: As needed until the cause is confirmed and treatment is adequate, effective, safe, and stable.

Maximum certification: 2 years

Certification recommendations:

✓ Certify if the history of seizures is limited to childhood febrile seizures.

✗ Do not certify if the examiner believes that the nature and severity of the driver's medical condition endangers the health and safety of the driver and the public.

Follow-up: At least biennial medical exams (every 2 years)

4. Epilepsy

Epilepsy is a chronic functional disease characterized by seizures or episodes that occur without warning, resulting in loss of voluntary control which may lead to loss of consciousness and/or seizures. Therefore, a driver cannot be qualified if he or she:

• Has a medical history of epilepsy,

• Has a current clinical diagnosis of epilepsy, or

• Is taking anti-seizure medication.

VI. Qualification Standards

Following an initial unprovoked seizure, the driver should be seizure free and off anticonvulsant medication for at least 5 years to distinguish between a "medical history of a single instance of seizure" and epilepsy. A second unprovoked seizure, regardless of the elapsed time between seizures, is a "medical history of epilepsy" and the driver would no longer meet the physical requirements under §391.41(b)(8).

> **NOTE:** Epilepsy medical guidelines are currently under review. While there have been no changes to the wording of §391.41(b)(8), current advisory criteria allow that some "drivers with a history of epilepsy/seizures [who are] off antiseizure medication and seizure-free for 10 years may be qualified to drive a CMV in interstate commerce."

Waiting period before certification: At least 10 years after being taken off anticonvulsant medication and free of seizures.

Certification recommendations:

✓ Certify if the driver has completed a waiting period of 10 years off anticonvulsant medication and seizure free, and the examiner believes the driver can safely drive.

✗ Do not certify (based on federal regulations) if the driver has:

- An established medical history of epilepsy,

- A clinical diagnosis of epilepsy, or

- Any other condition likely to cause loss of consciousness or any loss of ability to control a CMV.

✗ Do not certify (based on recommendations) if the driver is taking anticonvulsant medication because of a medical history of one or more seizures or is at risk for seizures.

NOTE: If the examiner chooses to certify a driver with an established medical history of epilepsy, the examiner must document support for that decision.

Monitoring/testing: Clearance from a specialist in neurological diseases is recommended if the examiner chooses to certify a driver with an established history of epilepsy.

Follow-up: Annual medical exams

5. Headaches

Chronic headaches can potentially lead to other neurological complications, such as stroke in relation to migraines, or have other symptoms of their own, like the visual distortion or loss of equilibrium associated with a migraine attack.

The following types of headaches may interfere with the ability to safely drive a CMV:

- Migraines,
- Tension-type headaches,
- Cluster headaches,
- Post-traumatic head-injury syndrome,
- Headaches associated with substances or withdrawal,
- Cranial neuralgias, and
- Atypical facial pain.

Examiners will consider headache frequency and severity when evaluating a driver whose history includes headaches. Other symptoms caused by headaches besides pain, such as visual disturbances, may interfere with safe driving as well. Examiners will also consider the effects of treatment used to relieve headaches.

Waiting period before certification: As needed until the cause is confirmed and treatment is adequate, effective, safe, and stable.

Maximum certification: 2 years

STANDARDS

Certification recommendations:

✗ <u>Do not certify</u> if the driver's medical condition endangers the health and safety of the driver and the public.

Follow-up: Biennial medical exams (every 2 years)

6. Single Unprovoked Seizure

An unprovoked seizure occurs without an identifiable systemic illness or brain injury, although the cause may be known and/or distant.

While individuals who experience a single unprovoked seizure do not have a diagnosis of epilepsy, they are clearly at a higher risk for having further seizures. The overall occurrence rate is estimated to be 36% within the first 5 years following the seizure. After 5 years, the risk for recurrence is down to 2% to 3% per year on average.

Following an initial unprovoked seizure, the driver should be seizure free and off anticonvulsant medication for at least 5 years to distinguish between a "medical history of a single unprovoked seizure" and epilepsy (two or more unprovoked seizures). A second unprovoked seizure, regardless of the elapsed time between seizures, would be a "medical history of epilepsy," and the driver would no longer meet the physical requirements for §391.41(b)(8).

The length of time an individual is seizure free and off anticonvulsant medication is considered the best predictor of future risk for seizures. Therefore, for the entire waiting period before being considered for certification, the driver should be both seizure free and off anticonvulsant medication prescribed for control of seizures.

Waiting period before certification: At least 5 years seizure free and off anticonvulsant medication.

Maximum certification: 1 year

Certification recommendations:

✓ <u>Certify</u> if the waiting period has passed and the driver has clearance from a neurologist who specializes in epilepsy and understands the demands of commercial driving.

Follow-up: Biennial medical exams (every 2 years)

7. Vertigo and Dizziness

The normal ability to maintain balance and orientation while driving a CMV depends on coordinated effort by the peripheral and central nervous systems. Inappropriate interactions of these systems or interactions within the nervous system may produce an unsafe degree of vertigo or dizziness.

The most common medications used to treat vertigo are antihistamines, benzodiazepines, and phenothiazines.

➤ **Use of either benzodiazepines or phenothiazines for the treatment of vertigo would make the driver medically unqualified.**

Antihistamines have possible sedative side effects, which should be taken into consideration for CMV drivers.

Waiting period before certification: At least 2 months symptom-free with diagnosis of benign positional vertigo or acute and chronic peripheral vestibulopathy.

Maximum certification: 2 years; or 1 year for any driver who requires special evaluation and screening.

Certification recommendations:

✓ Certify if the waiting period has passed and the nature and severity of the driver's medical condition do not endanger public safety.

✗ Do not certify if:
- The waiting period has not passed; or
- The driver has a diagnosis of Meniere's disease, Labyrinthine fistula, or non-functioning labyrinths.

Follow-up: Biennial medical exams (every 2 years)

Infections of the Central Nervous System

The guidelines for central nervous system (CNS) infection consider diagnosis and whether or not the driver has a history of early seizures with the condition. Aseptic meningitis is not associated with any increase in seizure risk, so no restrictions should be considered for drivers with such a condition.

A driver with a current clinical CNS diagnosis or signs and symptoms of a CNS infection should not be considered for certification until the cause is confirmed and treatment is adequate, effective, safe, and stable.

Waiting period before certification:

If seizure free and off anticonvulsant medication following:	Then wait at least:
• Bacterial meningitis without early seizures, or • Viral encephalitis without early seizures	1 year
Bacterial meningitis with early seizures	5 years
Viral encephalitis with early seizures	10 years

Maximum certification: 2 years

Certification recommendations:

 Certify if the driver has a history of:
- Aseptic meningitis,
- Bacterial meningitis (after waiting period has passed), or
- Viral encephalitis (after waiting period has passed).

✗ Do not certify if the driver has a current CNS infection.

Follow-up: Annual medical exams may be appropriate

Neuromuscular Diseases

Neuromuscular diseases develop slowly, generally measured in months to years. Rare neuromuscular diseases may be episodic producing weakness over minutes to hours.

The examiner will consider the effects of neuromuscular conditions on the driver's physical ability to drive, including steering, braking, clutching, getting in and out of vehicles, and reaction time. The examiner may order additional assessment from a neurologist or physiatrist.

1. Autonomic Neuropathy

Autonomic neuropathy affects the nerves that regulate vital functions, including the heart muscle and other muscles.

Waiting period before certification: As needed until the cause is confirmed and treatment is adequate, effective, safe, and stable.

Maximum certification: 2 years

VI. *Qualification Standards*

Certification recommendations:

✓ Certify if the medical condition does not endanger public safety.

✗ Do not certify if the driver has:
  • Cardiovascular autonomic neuropathy that causes resting tachycardia or orthostatic blood pressure, or

  • Other organ autonomic neuropathy that interferes with driving ability.

Follow-up: Biennial medical exams (every 2 years), or as needed for adequate monitoring

2. Conditions Associated With Abnormal Muscle Activity

This group of disorders is characterized by abnormal muscle excitability caused by abnormalities either in the nerve or in the muscle membrane.

Waiting period before certification: As needed until the cause is confirmed and treatment is adequate, effective, safe, and stable.

Maximum certification: 2 years

Certification recommendations:

✓ Certify if the driver's condition does not endanger public safety.

✗ Do not certify if the driver has a diagnosis of myotonia, Isaac's syndrome, or stiff-man syndrome.

Follow-up: Biennial medical exams (every 2 years), or as needed for adequate monitoring

3. Other Neuromuscular Diseases

Drivers who are diagnosed with the following neuromuscular diseases may NOT be certified. However, see "NOTE" below.

DISEASE	DESCRIPTION
Congenital myopathies	Congenital myopathies (muscle diseases that are present at birth) are a group of disorders that may be distinguished from others because of specific, well-defined structural alterations of the muscle fiber and may be progressive or non-progressive. These disorders include: • Central core disease, • Centronuclear myopathy, • Congenital muscular dystrophy, and • Rod (nemaline) myopathy. Inflammatory myopathies are acquired muscle diseases that may be treated. These disorders include dermatomyositis, inclusion body myositis, and polymyositis.
Metabolic muscle diseases	Metabolic muscle diseases are a group of disorders comprised of conditions affecting the energy metabolism of muscle or an imbalance in the chemical composition either within or surrounding the muscle. Conditions may affect glycogen and glycolytic metabolism, lipid metabolism, mitochondrial metabolism, or potassium balance of the muscle. Unlike most other neuromuscular disorders, these conditions may either progress slowly or be episodic.
Motor neuron diseases	This group of disorders includes: • Hereditary spinal muscular atrophy in both juvenile and adult forms; and • Acquired amyotrophic lateral sclerosis conditions producing degeneration of the motor nerve cells in the spinal cord. As a group, these are debilitating, progressive conditions that interfere with the ability to drive commercial vehicles.
Muscular dystrophies	Muscular dystrophies are hereditary, progressive, degenerative diseases of the muscle that interfere with safe driving.

DISEASE	DESCRIPTION
Neuromuscular junction disorders	This group of disorders includes myasthenia gravis and myasthenic syndrome. In addition to limb-muscle weakness, vision is often affected and sufferers are often easily fatigued.
Peripheral neuropathies	This group of disorders consists of hereditary and acquired conditions where sensory and/or motor nerves are affected, and may be a complication of diabetes.

NOTE: Neuromuscular disorders represent a complex group of conditions. The severity can vary with the individual and in certain instances may be treatable or non-progressive.

The decision not to certify a driver may be reconsidered if the driver is evaluated by a neurologist or physiatrist who understands the demands of commercial driving. The specialist may recommend a simulated driving skills test or equivalent functional test. When appropriate, the driver may need annual recertification with annual evaluation by a specialist and annual driving tests.

Progressive Neurological Conditions

Guidelines recommend that any driver having neurological signs or symptoms be referred to a neurologist for a more detailed evaluation. The specialist must understand the role, function, and demands of a CMV driver.

1. Central Nervous System Tumors

The central nervous system (CNS) is the seat of our intelligence and emotions, and an affliction of the CNS impacts everyday functioning in a direct and visible way. Brain tumors may alter cognitive abilities and judgment, and these symptoms may occur early in the course of the condition. Sensory and motor abnormalities may be produced both by brain tumors and by spinal cord tumors, depending on the location.

For some benign tumors, certification may be possible after successful surgical treatment.

The length of time an individual is seizure free and off of anticonvulsant medication is considered the best predictor of future risk for seizures. Therefore, for the entire waiting period before being considered for certification, the driver must be both seizure free and off anticonvulsant medication prescribed for control of seizures.

Waiting period before certification:

After surgical removal of:	the minimum waiting period is:
• Infratentorial meningiomas, • Acoustic neuromas, • Pituitary adenomas, • Spinal benign tumors, or • Benign extra-axial tumors	1 year.
• Benign supratentorial tumors, or • Spinal tumors	2 years.

Maximum certification: 1 year

Certification recommendations:

 Certify if the driver has:
  • Completed the appropriate minimum waiting period,
  • Stable non-progressive deficit or no neurological deficit, and
  • Imaging that shows no tumors.

✗ Do not certify if the driver has:
  • Not completed the waiting period,
  • Primary or metastatic malignant tumors of the nervous system, or
  • Benign nervous system tumors.

> **NOTE:** If the driver has a history of seizures, the appropriate seizure guidelines should be followed.

Monitoring/testing: Residual exams must show no evidence of recurrent or new tumors. Evaluation should be performed by a neurologist or physiatrist who understands the demands of commercial driving.

Follow-up: Annual medical exams

2. Dementia

Dementia is a progressive decline in mental functioning that can interfere with memory, language, spatial functions, higher-order perceptual functions, problem solving, judgment, behavior, and emotional functions. Alzheimer's and Pick's diseases both cause dementia and have symptoms that may lead to unsafe driving. Neither disease has a specific diagnostic test, with mild symptoms typically present for years before the diagnosis is made. Alzheimer's is the most common degenerative disease.

✗ Drivers diagnosed with dementia should <u>not</u> be certified because:
  - There is no current evidence that a driver diagnosed with dementia can safely drive a CMV, and
  - The disease progresses at a variable rate.

Static Neurological Conditions

Static neurological conditions include common cerebrovascular disease, as well as head and spinal cord injuries.

Cerebrovascular events may cause cognitive, judgment, attention, concentration, and/or motor and sensory impairments that can interfere with normal and safe driving. Drivers with several types of cerebrovascular disease are also at risk for recurring events that can happen without warning. Drivers with ischemic cerebrovascular disease are also at high risk for acute cardiac events, including heart attacks or sudden death. Recurrent cerebrovascular symptoms or cardiac events can occur with sufficient frequency to cause concern about the safe operation of a CMV.

The common types of cerebrovascular disease are:

- Transient ischemic attack/minor stroke with minimal or no lasting impairment;

- Embolic or thrombotic cerebral infarction with moderate to major lasting impairment; and

- Intracerebral or subarachnoid hemorrhage.

Drivers with head injuries are to have a complete physical exam, neurological exam, and neuropsychological testing. If results are normal, then certification is based on the seizure guidelines. Spinal cord injury resulting in paraplegia is disqualifying. Any weakness should be evaluated to determine whether it interferes with the job requirements of a commercial driver.

Any driver with a neurological deficit that requires special evaluation and screening should have annual medical exams.

1. Embolic and Thrombotic Strokes

More than 3 million individuals have survived a stroke, a major cause of long-term disability. Embolic and thrombotic cerebral infarctions are the most common forms of cardiovascular disease. Risk for complicating seizures is associated with the location of the lesions. Cerebellum and brainstem vascular lesions are not associated with an increased risk for seizures, but cortical and subcortical deficits are.

Evaluation by a neurologist is necessary to confirm the area of involvement.

Drivers with embolic or thrombotic cerebral infarctions will have lasting intellectual or physical impairments. Fatigue, prolonged work, and stress may exaggerate the lasting neurological effects of a stroke. Most recovery from a stroke will occur within one year of the event.

Waiting period before certification: At least 1 year if not at risk for seizures (cerebellum or brainstem vascular lesions); at least 5 years if at risk for seizures (cortical or subcortical deficits).

Maximum certification: 1 year

Certification recommendations:

Certify if a driver with a history of stroke has:
- Completed the appropriate waiting period;

- A normal physical exam, neurological exam including neuro-ophthalmological evaluation, and neuropsychological testing;

- No lasting neurological effects or, if present, effects that do not interfere with safe driving; and

- Clearance from a neurologist who understands the demands of commercial driving.

Do not certify if the driver:
- Has not completed the appropriate waiting period;

- Uses oral anticoagulant therapy (due to risk of excessive bleeding);

- Uses any other drug(s) with potentially high rates of complications (e.g., depressing effects on the nervous system);

- Has lasting intellectual or physical impairments that interfere with commercial driving; and/or

- Does not have clearance from a neurologist.

Follow-up: Annual medical exams

2. Intracerebral and Subarachnoid Hemorrhages

Intracerebral hemorrhage results from bleeding into the substance of the brain and subarachnoid hemorrhage reflects bleeding primarily into the spaces around the brain. Bleeding occurs as a result of a number of conditions including hypertension, hemorrhagic disorders, trauma, cerebral aneurysms, neoplasms, arteriovenous malformations, and degenerative or inflammatory vasculopathies.

These hemorrhages can cause serious harm to cognitive abilities, judgment, attention, and physical skills.

Cerebellum and brainstem vascular hemorrhages are not associated with an increased risk for seizures, but cortical and subcortical hemorrhages are. Evaluation by a neurologist is required to confirm the area of involvement.

The recommendations for intracranial and subarachnoid hemorrhages parallel recommendations for strokes.

Waiting period before certification: At least 1 year if not at risk for seizures; at least 5 years if at risk for seizures.

Maximum certification: 1 year

Certification recommendations:

 Certify if the driver has:
- Completed the appropriate waiting period;
- A normal physical exam, neurological exam including neuro-ophthalmological evaluation, and neuropsychological testing;
- No lasting neurological effects or, if present, effects that do not interfere with safe driving; and
- Clearance from a neurologist who understands the demands of commercial driving.

✗ Do not certify if the driver:
- Has not completed the appropriate waiting period;
- Uses oral anticoagulant therapy (due to risk of excessive bleeding);
- Uses any other drug(s) with potentially high rates of complications (e.g., depressing effects on the nervous system);
- Has lasting intellectual or physical impairments that interfere with commercial driving; and/or
- Does not have clearance from a neurologist.

Follow-up: Annual medical exams

3. Transient Ischemic Attack

A transient ischemic attack (TIA), sometimes called a "mini stroke," is an episode of focal neurological dysfunction caused by inadequate blood supply to a portion of the brain. The attack usually lasts more than a few seconds but less than 20 minutes. In exceptional cases, the symptoms can persist for up to 24 hours.

Drivers who have suffered a TIA usually appear normal during a physical exam. However, a TIA episode is an important warning for a potentially severe stroke or other vascular event. The risk of recurrent events is highest during the first few weeks and months following the TIA, declining by year 1 to less than 5% per year. The risk of recurrent strokes may be lowered by medical or surgical interventions.

The medical examiner will determine certification on a case-by-case basis considering the interval history, general health, neurological exam, and compliance with the treatment program.

Waiting period before certification: At least 1 year

Maximum certification: 1 year

Certification recommendations:

 Certify if the driver has:

- Completed the minimum waiting period seizure free and off anticonvulsant medication;

- A normal physical exam, neurological exam including neuro-ophthalmological evaluation, and neuropsychological test; and

- Clearance from a neurologist who understands the demands of commercial driving.

X Do not certify if the driver uses:

- Oral anticoagulant therapy (due to risk of excess bleeding), or

- Any other drug(s) with a potentially high rate of complications (e.g., depressing effects on the nervous system).

Follow-up: Annual medical exams

STANDARDS

235

4. Traumatic Brain Injury

Traumatic brain injury (TBI) is an injury to the brain caused by an external physical force, which may produce a diminished or altered state of consciousness, including coma, resulting in long-term impairment of cognitive or physical function.

Disturbances of behavioral or emotional functioning may result in total or partial disability and/or psychological maladjustment. Many people with TBI suffer loss of memory and reasoning ability, experience speech and/or language problems, and exhibit emotional and behavioral changes that are medically disqualifying for commercial driving.

TBI is classified by depth of dural penetration (the tissue surrounding the brain) and duration of loss of consciousness. The three classes are:

- **Severe head injury** — Penetrates the dura and causes a loss of consciousness lasting longer than 24 hours. There is a high risk for unprovoked seizures, and the risk does not diminish over time.

- **Moderate head injury** — Does not penetrate the dura but causes a loss of consciousness lasting longer than 30 minutes, but less than 24 hours.

- **Mild head injury** — Has no dural penetration or loss of consciousness and lasts for fewer than 30 minutes.

The length of time an individual is seizure free and off anticonvulsant medication is considered the best predictor of future risk for seizures. Therefore, for the entire waiting period before being considered for certification, the driver must be both seizure free and off anticonvulsant medication prescribed for control of seizures.

> **NOTE:** Surgical procedures involving dural penetration have a risk for subsequent epilepsy similar to that of severe head trauma. Individuals who have undergone such procedures, including those who have had surgery for epilepsy, should not be considered eligible for certification.

Waiting period before certification: At least 2 years seizure free and off anticonvulsant medication following:

- Moderate TBI without early seizures, or

- Mild TBI with early seizures.

At least 5 years seizure free and off anticonvulsant medication following moderate TBI with early seizures.

Maximum certification: 1 year; or 2 years for mild TBI without early seizures

Certification recommendations:

✓ Certify if the driver with a mild or moderate TBI has:
  - Completed the minimum waiting period;
  - A normal physical exam, neurological exam including neuro-ophthalmological evaluation, and neuropsychological test; and
  - Clearance from a neurologist who understands the demands of commercial driving.

✗ Do not certify if the driver has sustained a severe TBI, with or without early seizures.

Follow-up: Annual medical exams

Summary of Neurological Waiting Periods

Seizure waiting periods

Diagnosis	Waiting Period*
• History of epilepsy, or • Viral encephalitis with early seizures	10 years
• Single unprovoked seizure, no identified acute change, may be distant cause (possible earlier return to driving if normal neurological exam by a specialist in epilepsy and the driver has a normal electroencephalogram); or • Bacterial meningitis and early seizures	5 years
Acute seizure with acute structural central nervous system injury	2 years
Acute seizure with acute systemic/metabolic illness	Based on risk of recurrence of primary condition

*Seizure-free and off anticonvulsant medication.

Other waiting periods

Diagnosis	Waiting Period*
• Moderate traumatic brain injury (TBI) with early seizures, • Stroke with risk for seizures, or • Intracerebral or subarachnoid hemorrhage with risk for seizures	5 years
• Moderate TBI without early seizures, or • Surgically removed supratentorial or spinal tumors	2 years
• Transient ischemic attack, stroke, or intracerebral or subarachnoid hemorrhages with no risk for seizures; • Surgically-repaired arteriovenous malformations/aneurysm with no risk for seizures; • Surgically removed infratentorial meningiomas, acoustic neuromas, pituitary adenomas, and benign spinal tumors or other benign extraaxial tumors with no risk for seizures; or • Infections of the central nervous system (e.g., bacterial meningitis, viral encephalitis without early seizures)	1 year

*Seizure-free and off anticonvulsant medication.

Musculoskeletal

The standard: §391.41(b)(1), (2), (7)

A person is physically qualified to drive a commercial motor vehicle (CMV) if that person has no:

- Loss of a foot, leg, hand, or arm;

- Impairment of:

  - A hand or finger which interferes with grasping; or

  - An arm, foot, or leg which interferes with the ability to perform normal CMV-related tasks;

- Other significant limb defect or limitation which interferes with the ability to perform normal CMV-related tasks; or

- Established history or diagnosis of rheumatic, arthritic, orthopedic, muscular, neuromuscular, or vascular disease which interferes with safe driving.

In some cases, drivers may be certified if they are able to obtain a Skill Performance Evaluation certificate under §391.49

Public safety considerations:

Disorders of the musculoskeletal system affect driving ability and functionality necessary to perform heavy-labor tasks associated with the job of commercial driving. Medical certification means the driver is physically able to safely drive and perform non-driving tasks, from loading, unloading, and securing cargo to shifting gears, braking, and performing vehicle inspections.

The exam:

The examiner must determine whether the driver has the musculoskeletal strength, flexibility, dexterity, and balance to maintain control of the vehicle and safely perform non-driving tasks. The examiner will adapt the exam to cover the physical demands of driving, e.g., rotation of the outstretched arms against resistance as if turning a large steering wheel, movement of the legs in braking and clutching, etc.

Examiners will evaluate and/or ask about diseases, limb impairments, spinal injuries, weakness or tenderness, lower-back pain, limping, medications, etc. The examiner may order radiological, neurological, or other exams as necessary.

Fixed Deficit of an Extremity

When the loss of a hand, foot, leg, or arm or a permanent impairment to an extremity may interfere with the ability to drive safely, the driver may be allowed to drive if the qualification requirements for a Skill Performance Evaluation (SPE) certificate under §391.49 are met.

The driver may be able to safely operate a CMV by use of technology, medical aids, and/or equipment modifications.

In order to legally operate a CMV, the driver must carry:

• An SPE certificate, AND

• A valid medical examiner's certificate.

The driver is responsible for ensuring that both certificates are renewed prior to expiration.

Waiting period before certification: The driver must be otherwise medically fit for duty before certification under the SPE program.

Maximum certification period: 2 years

Certification recommendations:

 Certify if the driver has:
- A permanent impairment to an extremity but is otherwise medically qualified; and

- A valid SPE certificate at recertification, and documentation of compliance with medical requirements.

✗ Do not certify if the driver has:
- An impairment that affects the torso;

- Not provided proof of compliance with SPE certification requirements; or

- A disqualifying limb impairment caused by a progressive disease (e.g., multiple sclerosis).

> **NOTE:** The SPE applies only to "fixed deficits" (permanent impairment) of the extremities, not those caused by a progressive disease.

Monitoring/testing: SPE applications (both initial and renewal) require a medical evaluation summary completed by either a board-qualified or board-certified physiatrist or orthopedic surgeon.

Follow-up: At least biennial physical exams (every 2 years)

Musculoskeletal Tests

Detection of an undiagnosed musculoskeletal finding during the physical exam may indicate the need for further testing and examination. Diagnostic-specific testing may be required to detect the presence and/or severity of the musculoskeletal condition. The additional testing may be ordered by the medical examiner, primary care physician, or musculoskeletal specialist (e.g., orthopedic surgeon, physiatrist). The specialist must understand the role and function of a CMV driver.

STANDARDS

241

Grip-Strength Tests

The FMCSA does not require any specific test for assessing grip power. Examples of grip-strength tests include:

- Dynamometer testing designed to measure grip strength; or

- Sphygmomanometer testing used as a screening test for grip by having the applicant repeatedly squeeze the inflated cuff while noting the maximum deflection on the gauge.

The driver must have sufficient grasp to control an oversize steering wheel, shift gears using a manual transmission, and maneuver a vehicle in crowded areas.

Obtaining and Using an SPE Certificate

Drivers who have lost a limb or suffer from limb impairment may only operate commercial vehicles in interstate commerce if they first obtain a Skill Performance Evaluation (SPE) certificate.

The requirements for obtaining the certificate are found in §391.49.

The underlying cause of the deficiency (e.g., trauma, cerebral palsy, or a birth defect) does not affect eligibility to apply for an SPE certificate. However, the location of the deficit must be an extremity, not the neck or torso.

NOTE: SPE certificates are issued for the operation of power units only. The employing motor carrier must evaluate the driver with a road test using the trailer type(s) the motor carrier intends the driver to transport, or the carrier may accept the trailer road test done during the SPE application process if it is a similar trailer type(s). The carrier must also evaluate the driver for non-driving, safety-related job tasks associated with the type(s) of trailer(s) used, as well as any other tasks unique to the carrier's operations.

The following are the basic steps needed to apply for an SPE certificate. These may be performed by an individual driver alone or with assistance from a motor carrier:

1. Be evaluated by a physiatrist (doctor of physical medicine) or orthopedic surgeon, providing him or her with a description of the job-related tasks the driver will be required to perform. Obtain a written medical evaluation.

2. Undergo a DOT medical exam and obtain a medical certificate. The certificate will indicate that an SPE certificate is required.

3. Complete a driver employment application or obtain a copy of the last driver application that was completed.

4. Obtain a driving record from the driver's licensing state covering the past three years.

5. Perform a road test, administered by a motor carrier or competent individual, and document the results according to §391.31.

6. Submit a letter of application for an SPE certificate to the FMCSA, including:

   • The information listed in §391.49(c),

   • A copy of the Medical Examination Report form with the "Skill Performance Evaluation (SPE) Certificate" box marked,

- A copy of the medical examiner's certificate indicating "accompanied by Skill Performance Evaluation Certificate (SPE),"

- The medical evaluation summary from the physiatrist or orthopedic surgeon,

- A description of any prosthetic or orthotic device being worn,

- A copy of the road test form,

- The driver application or a statement that the driver was not previously employed,

- A copy of any SPE certificate issued by the state, and

- The three-year driving record.

The SPE certificate is valid for up to 2 years and may be renewed 30 days prior to the expiration date.

> **NOTE:** Drivers licensed in the state of Virginia may be able to obtain an SPE certificate directly from the state, which has been authorized to issue certificates on behalf of the FMCSA. Contact the Virginia DMV for details.

Q: Does the driver need to carry the SPE certificate while on duty?
A: Yes. The driver must carry the SPE certificate or a legible copy at all times, even if (after January 2014) the driver is not required to carry the medical certificate. The driver is responsible for ensuring that both certificates are renewed prior to expiration.

Carrier Responsibilities

A motor carrier that hires a driver who carries an SPE certificate must:

- Notify the FMCSA in writing, within 30 days, of any accidents, arrests, convictions, or license/permit suspensions, revocations, or withdrawals involving the driver.

- Evaluate the driver with a road test using the trailer(s) the driver will be transporting, unless the carrier accepts a certificate of a trailer road test done by another motor carrier or during the SPE application process.

- Evaluate the driver for all non-driving, safety-related tasks that the driver will be performing.

- Use the driver to operate only the type of vehicle defined in the SPE certificate, and only when the driver is in compliance with the conditions and limitations of the certificate.

See §391.49 in Chapter 9 for complete requirements.

Neuromuscular Diseases

See *Neurological* section of this chapter for information about the following neuromuscular diseases:

- Autonomic Neuropathy

- Conditions Associated with Abnormal Muscle Activity

- Congenital Myopathies

- Metabolic Muscle Diseases

- Motor Neuron Diseases

- Muscular Dystrophies

- Neuromuscular Junction Disorders

- Peripheral Neuropathies

Diabetes Mellitus

The standard: §391.41(b)(3)

A person is physically qualified to drive a commercial motor vehicle (CMV) if that person "has no established medical history or clinical diagnosis of diabetes mellitus currently treated with insulin for control, unless the person meets the requirements in §391.46."

 Key points:

- Though the use of insulin can be disqualifying, simply being diagnosed with diabetes is not.

- If diabetes can be controlled through oral medication and diet, the driver may be certified.

- Drivers taking insulin can be certified under the process described in §391.46.

Public safety considerations:

Almost 24 million people in the U.S. (8% of the population) have diabetes, including about 18 million people who have been diagnosed and another 6 million who have not.

The most common form of diabetes is Type 2, also known as adult onset or non-insulin-dependent diabetes mellitus. Individuals with Type 2 diabetes can produce insulin and have intact blood glucose control, and may preserve that control for many years with lifestyle changes and oral hypoglycemic medications. Over time, however, their insulin production may fail, resulting in the need for insulin replacement therapy.

While managing both overly high and overly low blood-sugar levels are important aspects of diabetes management, hypoglycemia (unusually low levels of blood glucose) is more relevant to safety considerations for a diabetic driver.

- **Blood glucose control** — Some of the factors related to commercial driving that affect blood glucose control include fatigue, lack of sleep, poor diet, missed meals, emotional conditions, stress, and illness. These same factors may hasten the need for insulin therapy. Poorly controlled diabetes can result in serious, life-threatening health consequences. However, with good management of the disease process, a driver with diabetes can safely operate a CMV.

- **Hyperglycemia risk** — Poor blood glucose control can lead to fatigue, lethargy, and sluggishness. Complications related to acute hyperglycemia (unusually high blood-glucose levels) may affect driving ability. Complications can lead to medical conditions severe enough to be disqualifying, such as neuropathy, retinopathy, and nephropathy. Accelerated atherosclerosis (hardening of the arteries) is a major complication of diabetes involving the coronary, cerebral, and peripheral vessels. Individuals with diabetes are at increased risk for coronary heart disease and have a higher incidence of painless heart attacks than individuals who do not have diabetes.

- **Hypoglycemia risk** — Preventing hypoglycemia (unusually low blood-glucose levels) is the most critical and challenging safety issue for any driver with diabetes. Hypoglycemia can occur in individuals with diabetes who both use and do not use insulin. Mild hypoglycemia causes rapid heart rate, sweating, weakness, and hunger. Severe hypoglycemia can cause symptoms that interfere with safe driving.

The FMCSA defines a severe hypoglycemic reaction as one that results in:

- Seizure,

- Loss of consciousness,

- The need for assistance from another person, and/or

- Periods of impaired cognitive function that occur without warning.

The exam:

The medical examiner must determine whether the driver is at an unacceptable risk for sudden death or incapacitation, thus endangering public safety. The risk may be associated with the disease and/or the treatment.

The examiner has to determine if the driver has diabetes or elevated blood glucose controlled by diet, pills, insulin, or other injectable medications.

The examiner may also look into whether the driver is monitoring blood glucose, uses medications or supplements, has a history of fainting or dizziness, or a history of hypoglycemic reactions. If any hypoglycemic reactions have been severe, the examiner will look at the 5-year history of such reactions.

Diabetes Mellitus

A driver with diabetes mellitus who does NOT use insulin is eligible for certification, unless the driver also has a disqualifying complication, multiple illnesses, or fails to meet one or more of the other standards for qualification.

Though the healthcare provider treating the driver's diabetes is primarily concerned with minimizing target organ damage, the critical issue for the DOT medical examiner is assessing the driver for risk of a severe hypoglycemic episode.

Waiting period before certification: As needed until treatment is adequate, effective, safe, and stable.

Maximum certification: 2 years

> **NOTE:** For a driver diagnosed with diabetes, the FMCSA says annual certification is "reasonable" because of the progressive nature of diabetes.

Certification recommendations:

 Certify if the driver:
  - Meets all the physical qualification standards, and

  - Has a treatment plan that manages the disease and does not include the use of insulin or interfere with safe driving.

✘ Do not certify if the driver has:
  - In the last 12 months, experienced a hypoglycemic reaction resulting in seizure, loss of consciousness, need for assistance from another person, or a period of impaired cognitive function that occurred without warning;

  - In the last 5 years, had recurring (two or more) disqualifying hypoglycemic reactions;

  - Loss of position sensation;

  - Loss of sensation in the feet;

  - Resting tachycardia (rapid heart rate);

  - Orthostatic hypotension; or

  - A diagnosis of peripheral neuropathy or proliferative retinopathy (e.g., unstable proliferative or non-proliferative).

249

Monitoring/testing: Poor blood glucose control may be indicated by urinalysis showing sugar in the urine (glycosuria) or blood testing showing hemoglobin A1c (HbA1c) greater than 10%.

Follow-up: At least biennial exams (every 2 years)

> NOTE: Drivers with diabetes are encouraged to participate in annual diabetes education.

Incretin Mimetic Therapy

Non-insulin, anti-diabetic drugs known as "incretin mimetics," such as exenatide (Byetta), are used to improve glycemic control in people with Type 2 diabetes by reducing fasting and after-meal glucose concentrations. An incretin mimetic is typically taken in combination with other oral agents such as metformin. Use of an incretin mimetic in conjunction with drugs that increase insulin levels (e.g., sulfonylurea) lead to an increased risk of hypoglycemia.

➤ **Incretin mimetics are not insulin and can be used without any type of exemption.**

Waiting period before certification: As necessary until the treatment has been shown to be adequate, effective, safe, and stable.

Maximum certification: 1 year

> NOTE: The FMCSA recommends frequent monitoring determined on a case-by-case basis.

Certification recommendations:

 Certify if the driver:
- Meets all the physical qualification standards; and

- Has a treatment plan that manages the disease and does not include the use of insulin or have side effects that interfere with safe driving.

✗ Do not certify if the driver's condition and/or treatment endangers public safety.

Monitoring/testing: FMCSA recommends that drivers taking an incretin mimetic provide a written statement from their treating healthcare professional to their DOT medical examiner describing the driver's tolerance to the medication, how frequently the driver is monitored, and the effectiveness of treatment.

Follow-up: "Frequent" monitoring while the driver is taking an incretin mimetic.

Insulin Therapy

Diabetic drivers who need insulin for control of blood glucose levels also have treatment conditions that can be harmed by the use of too much or too little insulin, or food intake that is not consistent with the insulin dosage. The administration of insulin is a complicated process requiring insulin, syringe, needle, alcohol sponge, and a sterile technique. Factors related to long-haul driving, such as fatigue, lack of sleep, poor diet, emotional conditions, stress, and illness, compound the dangers.

The FMCSA has historically held that drivers who take insulin cannot be certified without getting a special exemption. Effective November 19, 2018, however, such drivers may be certified for up to one year if they comply with §391.46 and are otherwise medically qualified.

VI. Qualification Standards

See "The Federal Certification Process for Drivers Using Insulin," below.

> **NOTE:** The certification process outlined in §391.46 replaces two older waiver/exemption programs for insulin-using drivers:
> - The "grandfathering" provision in §391.64, which originated in 1996, came to an end effective Nov. 19, 2019.
> - The diabetes exemption program, which began in 2003, was withdrawn on Feb. 21, 2019.

Hypoglycemia risk: Preventing hypoglycemia (overly low blood sugar) is the most critical and challenging safety issue for any driver with diabetes. Individuals who use insulin are at an increased risk for hypoglycemic reactions. A severe hypoglycemic reaction can result in seizure, loss of consciousness, the need for assistance, and/or a period of impaired cognitive function that occurs without warning.

A driver with diabetes treated with insulin who experiences a severe hypoglycemic episode after being physically certified to drive is prohibited from operating a commercial motor vehicle and must report the episode to, and be evaluated by, a treating clinician as soon as possible.

"Rescue" glucose: In some cases, hypoglycemia can be self-treated by the ingestion of at least 20 grams of glucose tablets or carbohydrates. Consuming "rescue" glucose or carbohydrates may avert a hypoglycemic reaction for less than a 2-hour period.

➤ **Drivers should be advised to carry a source of rapidly absorbable glucose while driving.**

Waiting period before certification: No specific waiting period is indicated. However, a driver must provide his/her treating clinician with 3 months' worth of electronic blood glucose self-monitoring records, while being treated with insulin, before he/she may be certified for 12 months.

Maximum certification: 1 year, or 3 months if the driver has not provided his/her treating clinician with at least the preceding 3 months' worth of electronic blood glucose self-monitoring records while being treated with insulin.

Certification recommendations:

 Certify if the driver:

- Meets all other physical qualification requirements except for the use of insulin;

- Was evaluated by his/her treating clinician and provides the medical examiner with form MCSA-5870 completed within the past 45 days; and

- Is free of complications from diabetes mellitus that might impair his/her ability to operate a commercial motor vehicle safely.

✕ Do not certify if the driver has:

- Any other medical problem or condition (other than the use of insulin) that prevents certification;

- Not maintained a stable insulin regimen;

- Not properly controlled his/her diabetes mellitus;

- Either severe non-proliferative diabetic retinopathy or proliferative diabetic retinopathy;

- Loss of position sensation;

- Loss of sensation in the feet;

- Resting tachycardia; or

- Orthostatic hypotension.

VI. Qualification Standards

Monitoring/testing:

- **Blood glucose monitoring** — The certification process outlined in §391.46 requires drivers to self-monitor blood glucose in accordance with a treatment plan prescribed by the treating clinician. Such drivers must maintain blood glucose records measured with an electronic glucometer that stores all readings, that records the date and time of readings, and from which data can be electronically downloaded. Drivers must provide a printout of their electronic blood glucose records, or the glucometer itself, to the treating clinician at the time of any required evaluations. The treating clinician must then complete FMCSA form MCSA-5870 and provide a copy to the driver to bring to a medical examiner within 45 days.

- **Urinalysis** — Poor blood glucose control may be indicated by urinalysis showing sugar in the urine (glycosuria).

- **Blood glucose** — Poor blood glucose control may indicate a need for further evaluation or more frequent monitoring.

> **NOTE:** Blood glucose levels that remain within the range of 100 to 400 mg/dL are generally considered safe for commercial driving.

Follow-up: At least annual exams.

Oral Hypoglycemics

Hypoglycemic drugs taken orally are frequently prescribed for persons with diabetes to help stimulate natural production of insulin. If diabetes can be controlled by the use of oral medication and diet, the driver may be considered for certification.

Waiting period before certification: As necessary until the treatment has been shown to be adequate, effective, safe, and stable.

Maximum certification: 1 year

Certification recommendations:

✓ <u>Certify</u> if the driver meets all the physical qualification standards and has a treatment plan that manages the disease and does not include the use of insulin or have side effects that interfere with safe driving.

✗ <u>Do not certify</u> if the driver's condition and/or treatment endangers public safety.

Follow-up: At least biennial exams (every 2 years)

The Federal Certification Process for Drivers Using Insulin

The FMCSA has transitioned to a new certification process for drivers with insulin-treated diabetes mellitus (ITDM). The process is described in §391.46, as found in the Reference chapter and summarized below.

➤ **Drivers with ITDM who are licensed in Canada or Mexico cannot operate in the United States and are not eligible for the certification process in §391.46.**

Grandfathering and Exemption Programs

In 2019, two programs that allowed drivers with ITDM to operate commercial vehicles in interstate commerce were phased out:

• On February 21, 2019, the FMCSA ended an exemption program that began in 2003. The program allowed some drivers with stable ITDM to become conditionally certified and then apply for a two-year exemption from the FMCSA.

255

- November 19, 2019, marks the end of the "grandfather" exemption under §391.64, which applied to a small number of drivers who had participated in a waiver study program in the mid-1990s.

Drivers who used either of the above programs must use the process in §391.46 to become re-certified at the time their current certifications expire.

> **NOTE:** Some states also issue waivers or exemptions from their diabetes standards for in-state drivers who are not subject to the federal standards. Drivers who have a state-issued diabetes exemption should notify their medical examiner.

Public Safety Considerations:

Type 1 diabetes accounts for 5-10% of all diagnosed cases of diabetes in adults. Individuals with type 1 diabetes have a virtual lack of insulin production, with associated complications, and must have insulin replacement therapy.

Although hypoglycemia (overly low blood sugar) can occur in non-insulin-treated diabetes, it is most often associated with insulin-treated diabetes. Mild hypoglycemia causes rapid heart rate, sweating, weakness, and hunger, while severe hypoglycemia causes headache and dizziness. The FMCSA defines a "severe" hypoglycemic reaction as one that requires the assistance of others or results in loss of consciousness, seizure, or coma. A driver who suffers a severe hypoglycemic reaction must stop driving and report to his/her treating clinician, as noted below.

Steps in the Certification Process

The following are the basic steps involved in certifying a driver with insulin-treated diabetes:

1. The driver must follow the treatment plan prescribed by his/her treating clinician, i.e., the state-licensed individual who prescribes the driver's

insulin and treatment plan. The driver must keep blood glucose records from an electronic glucometer that records the date and time of each reading (typed or handwritten logs are not allowed). Three months of records must be collected in order to obtain a 12-month certificate (anything less and the driver may only be certified for up to 3 months).

2. The driver must schedule a visit with the treating clinician and must bring along the glucometer or a printout of the electronic blood glucose records. The driver or treating clinician must also have a copy of the "Insulin-Treated Diabetes Mellitus Assessment Form" (MCSA-5870), available from the FMCSA.

3. The treating clinician must complete and sign the ITDM Assessment Form and provide the driver with a copy.

4. Within 45 days of the date the form was completed, the driver must obtain a medical exam from an examiner listed on the National Registry of Certified Medical Examiners. The driver must bring along the completed ITDM Assessment Form.

5. The medical examiner must use his/her independent clinical judgment to decide if the driver can be certified, and for how long, based on a complete medical exam and a review of the ITDM Assessment Form. The examiner must retain the form along with the medical examination report form.

6. The driver must repeat the above steps at least annually to remain certified.

If a driver is certified and later suffers a **severe hypoglycemic episode**, the driver must stop driving and must report the episode to his/her treating clinician as soon as possible. Before the individual may drive again, the clinician must:

• Determine that the cause of the severe hypoglycemic episode has been addressed;

- Determine that the driver is maintaining a stable insulin regimen and proper control of his/her diabetes; and

- Complete a new ITDM Assessment Form (MCSA-5870).

Certification Considerations

During the driver's medical examination, the examiner must:

- Review the ITDM Assessment Form and ensure that it was signed and dated within the past 45 days by the driver's treating clinician;

- Ensure that the driver is physically qualified in accordance with §391.43 and meets the physical qualification standards in §391.41, based on the examiner's independent medical judgment;

- Ensure that the driver is free of complications from diabetes mellitus that might impair his/her ability to operate a commercial motor vehicle safely; and

- Retain the completed ITDM Assessment Form for at least 3 years as part of the Medical Examination Report Form (MCSA-5875).

A driver is NOT physically qualified to operate a commercial motor vehicle if he/she:

- Is not maintaining a stable insulin regimen,

- Is not properly controlling his/her diabetes mellitus, or

- Has either severe non-proliferative diabetic retinopathy or proliferative diabetic retinopathy.

A driver who meets the conditions above may be certified for up to 12 months. However, if the driver does not give the treating clinician at least the preceding 3 months of electronic blood glucose self-monitoring records while being treated with insulin, the driver may be certified for no more than 3 months.

The Medical Certificate

When certifying a driver who uses insulin, the periodic monitoring interval shown on the Medical Examination Report form must:

- Agree with the Medical Examiner's Certificate expiration date, and

- Not exceed 1 year.

> ⊗ Meets standards, but periodic monitoring required *(specify reason):* __Insulin Use__
> Driver qualified for: ○ 3 months ○ 6 months ⊗ 1 year ○ other *(specify):* _____
> ☐ Wearing corrective lenses ☐ Wearing hearing aid ☐ Accompanied by a waiver/exemption *(specify type):* ____

NOTE: The examiner must NOT mark the "Accompanied by a _____ waiver/exemption" checkbox to note that a driver was certified under §391.46, because §391.46 does not involve a waiver or exemption program.

Other Diseases

The standard: §391.41(b)(9)

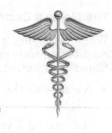

A person is physically qualified to drive a commercial motor vehicle (CMV) if that person "has no mental, nervous, organic, or functional disease or psychiatric disorder likely to interfere with his/her ability to drive a commercial motor vehicle safely."

Public safety considerations:

Examples of how medical conditions might interfere with safe driving:

- Emotional or adjustment problems contribute directly to an individual's level of memory, reasoning, attention, and judgment, and often underlie physical disorders.

- A variety of functional disorders can cause drowsiness, dizziness, confusion, weakness, or paralysis that may lead to incoordination, inattention, loss of functional control, and susceptibility to crashes while driving.

- Physical fatigue, headache, impaired coordination, recurring physical ailments, and chronic "nagging" pain may be present to such a degree that certification for commercial driving is inadvisable.

Nephropathy

Diabetic nephropathy, a disease of the kidneys, accounts for a significant number of kidney-disease cases. Protein in the urine is often the first sign of nephropathy, with end-stage renal disease following some time later. Whether nephropathy is disqualifying depends on how it's progressing and affecting the driver's ability to function.

The prevalence of nephropathy is strongly related to the duration of diabetes. After 15 years of living with diabetes, the frequency of nephropathy is higher among individuals who use insulin than with individuals who do not use insulin.

Waiting period before certification: As necessary until the cause is confirmed and treatment is adequate, effective, safe, and stable.

Maximum certification: 2 years

Certification recommendations:

 Certify if the driver:
- Meets all the physical qualification standards, and

- Has a treatment plan that manages the disease and does not interfere with safe driving.

Monitoring/testing: An abnormal urinalysis may indicate some degree of kidney dysfunction. The examiner may order additional tests and/or consultation as necessary.

Follow-up: At least biennial medical exams (every 2 years)

Hernia

Part of the physical exam involves checking for hernia for both the abdomen and viscera body system and the genitourinary system.

If a hernia causes discomfort or the diagnosis suggests that the condition might interfere with safe driving, further testing and evaluation may be required.

Waiting period before certification: As necessary until the cause is confirmed and treatment is adequate, effective, safe, and stable.

VI. *Qualification Standards*

Maximum certification: 2 years

Certification recommendations:

✔ <u>Certify</u> if the driver's condition does not endanger public safety.

Monitoring/testing: The examiner may order additional tests and/or consultation as needed.

Follow-up: At least biennial medical exams (every 2 years)

Psychological

The standard: §391.41(b)(9)

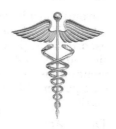

A person is physically qualified to drive a commercial motor vehicle (CMV) if that person "has no mental, nervous, organic, or functional disease or psychiatric disorder likely to interfere with his/her ability to drive a commercial motor vehicle safely."

Public safety considerations:

Safe and effective CMV operation requires high levels of physical strength, skill, and coordination as well as the ability to stay attentive and react promptly and appropriately to traffic, emergency situations, and other job-related stressors.

Some psychological or personality disorders can directly affect memory, reasoning, motor response, attention, and judgment, thus interfering with driving ability. The FMCSA recommends that somatic and psychosomatic complaints be thoroughly examined. Disorders of a periodically incapacitating nature, even in the early stages of development, may warrant disqualification.

Risk:

There are three categories of risk associated with psychological disorders and their effect on safe driving:

- The **mental disorder** itself, including symptoms and/or disturbances in performance;

- **Lingering symptoms** that may occur later; and

- **Medications** which can sometimes make driving hazardous.

Drivers diagnosed with a mental disorder are not automatically excluded from being certified. Typically, the more serious the diagnosis, the more likely it is that the driver will be medically disqualified.

Careful consideration is given to the side effects and interactions of medications. Many of the medications used to treat psychological disorders have effects and/or side effects that render driving unsafe. Medical recommendations use the degree of impairment produced by a 0.04 percent blood alcohol concentration as a benchmark.

The exam:

The medical examiner may investigate any psychological symptoms and order screening tests when indicated by the driver's affect, behavior, or interactions with the examiner.

The examiner should consider such factors as medication and alcohol use, severe depression and thoughts of suicide, inappropriate dress, suspiciousness, hostility or violence, unusual or bizarre ideas, hallucinations, dishonesty, or the omission of important information.

Adult ADHD

Children who had attention deficit hyperactivity disorder (ADHD) often continue to show signs of the disorder into adulthood. Features of adult ADHD include age-inappropriate levels of inattention, impulsiveness, and hyperactivity. Symptoms include mood swings, low frustration tolerance, and explosiveness.

Risks to safe driving associated with adult ADHD include antisocial or borderline personality disorder and/or other disorders, side effects of medication, and a high incidence of substance abuse. However, a significant percentage of individuals with adult ADHD show improvement on medications that stimulate the central nervous system.

Waiting period before certification: As necessary until the cause is confirmed and treatment is adequate, effective, safe, and stable.

Maximum certification: 1 year

Certification recommendations:

 Certify if the driver:
- Complies with the treatment program;

- Tolerates treatment without disqualifying side effects (e.g., sedation or impaired coordination); and

- Is evaluated by a mental health professional who understands the demands of commercial driving.

✗ Do not certify if the driver has:
- Active psychosis;

- Prominent negative symptoms including substantially compromised judgment, difficulty paying attention, suicidal behavior or ideas, or personality disorder that repeatedly leads to openly inappropriate acts; or

- Side effects that interfere with safe driving.

Monitoring/testing: The examiner may order additional tests and/or consult with a mental health specialist, such as a psychiatrist or psychologist, as necessary.

Follow-up: Annual medical exams

Central Nervous System Stimulant Therapy

Psychiatric uses of central nervous system (CNS) stimulants (e.g., dextroamphetamine, methylphenidate, and pemoline) include treatment of narcolepsy and adult attention deficit hyperactivity disorder (ADHD), both of which may lead to sleepiness or hyperactivity. CNS stimulants may also be used in combination with antidepressants.

For some conditions (e.g., fatigue, brain damage, adult ADHD), low doses of CNS stimulants can enhance vigilance, attention, and performance of simple tasks, but not complex intellectual functions.

Before a driver with ADHD who is using a CNS stimulant can be qualified, the examiner should verify the diagnosis, request evaluation from the treating healthcare provider, and use caution when determining the side effects of medication.

Waiting period before certification: As necessary until the medication is adequate, effective, safe, and stable.

Maximum certification: 1 year

Certification recommendations:

 Certify if the driver has:
- A non-disqualifying underlying condition (e.g., adult ADHD),
- No drug-induced impairment, and
- No tendency to increase the dose.

✗ Do not certify if the driver has:
- A disqualifying underlying condition (e.g., narcolepsy), or
- Treatment side effects that interfere with safe driving.

Monitoring/testing: The examiner may order additional tests and/or consult with a mental health specialist, such as a psychiatrist or psychologist.

Follow-up: Annual medical exams

STANDARDS

Bipolar Mood Disorder

Mood disorders can interfere with the ability to function socially and occupationally. The two major groups of mood disorders are bipolar and depressive disorders. Bipolar disorder is characterized by extreme mood swings, from great excitement to severe depression.

- **Manic episodes** — A manic (overly excited) episode may start suddenly or gradually. Symptoms include excessively elevated, expansive, or irritable moods, sometimes with delusions or hallucinations. During a manic episode, judgment is frequently diminished and there is an increased risk of substance abuse. Treatment for bipolar mania may include lithium and/or anticonvulsants to stabilize mood and antipsychotics when psychosis is present.

- **Depressive episodes** — Symptoms of a depressive episode include loss of interest and motivation, poor sleep, appetite disturbance, fatigue, poor concentration, and indecisiveness. A severe depression is characterized by psychosis, severe slowing of thought and movement, significant cognitive impairment (especially poor concentration and attention), and suicidal thoughts or behavior. In addition to the medication used to treat mania, antidepressants may be used to treat bipolar depression.

Other psychiatric disorders, including substance abuse, frequently coexist with bipolar disorder.

NOTE: Cyclothymia is a mild form of bipolar disorder that causes brief episodes of depression or elevated mood, but typically does not cause marked impairment. Treatment may include medication.

Waiting period before certification:

At least:	symptom free, following:
6 months	A non-psychotic major depression that is not accompanied by suicidal behavior.
1 year	• A severe depressive episode, • A suicide attempt, or • A manic episode.

Maximum certification: 1 year

Certification recommendations:

 Certify if the driver:
- Completes the waiting period;
- Complies with the treatment program;
- Tolerates treatment without disqualifying side effects; and
- Is evaluated by a mental health professional who understands the demands of commercial driving.

X Do not certify if the driver has:
- Active psychosis;
- Prominent negative symptoms, including substantially compromised judgment, difficulty paying attention, suicidal behavior or ideas, or personality disorder that repeatedly leads to openly inappropriate acts; or
- Treatment side effects that interfere with safe driving.

Monitoring/testing: At least every 2 years the driver with a history of a major mood disorder should have evaluation and clearance from a mental health specialist, such as a psychiatrist or psychologist, who understands the demands of commercial driving.

The driver should report any manic or severe major depressive episode within 30 days to the driver's employer, medical examiner, or appropriate healthcare professional, and should seek medical care.

Follow-up: Annual medical exams

Major Depression

Major depression consists of one or more depressive episodes that may alter mood, cognitive function, behavior, and physiology. Symptoms may include a depressed or irritable mood, loss of interest or pleasure, social withdrawal, appetite and sleep disturbance that lead to weight change and fatigue, restlessness and agitation or malaise, impaired concentration and memory, poor judgment, and suicidal thoughts or attempts. Hallucinations and delusions may also develop.

Most individuals with major depression will recover; however, some will relapse within 5 years. A significant percentage will commit suicide; the risk is the greatest within the first few years.

Many patients experience stressful events in the 6 months prior to the onset of depression. In addition to antidepressants, other drug therapy may include anxiolytics, antipsychotics, and lithium. Medication may prevent or shorten future episodes. Electroconvulsive therapy is also used to treat some cases of severe depression.

Waiting period before certification:

At least:	symptom free, following:
6 months	A non-psychotic major depression that is not accompanied by suicidal behavior.
1 year	• A severe depressive episode, • A suicide attempt, or • A manic episode.

269

VI. Qualification Standards

Maximum certification: 1 year

Certification recommendations:

✓ <u>Certify</u> if the driver:
- Completes the waiting period;
- Complies with the treatment program;
- Tolerates treatment without disqualifying side effects; and
- Is evaluated by a mental health professional who understands the demands of commercial driving.

✗ <u>Do not certify</u> if the driver has:
- Active psychosis;
- Prominent negative symptoms, including substantially compromised judgment, difficulty paying attention, suicidal behavior or ideas, or personality disorder that repeatedly leads to openly inappropriate acts; or
- Treatment side effects that interfere with safe driving.

Monitoring/testing: At least every 2 years the driver with a history of a major mood disorder should be evaluated and cleared for driving by a mental health specialist, such as a psychiatrist or psychologist, who understands the demands of commercial driving.

> The driver should report any manic or severe major depressive episode within 30 days to the driver's employer, medical examiner, or appropriate healthcare professional, and should seek medical care.

Follow-up: Annual medical exams.

STANDARDS

Personality Disorders

Any personality disorder characterized by excessive, aggressive, or impulsive behaviors should be investigated to determine if the individual is able to drive safely. A person is medically unqualified if the disorder is severe enough to have repeatedly interfered with safe driving.

> **NOTE:** Alcohol and drug dependency and abuse are profound risk factors in the presence of personality disorders.

Waiting period before certification: As necessary until the cause is confirmed and treatment is adequate, effective, safe, and stable.

Maximum certification: 1 year

Certification recommendations:

 Certify if the driver:
- Complies with treatment;
- Tolerates treatment without disqualifying side effects; and
- Is evaluated by a mental health professional who understands the demands of commercial driving.

✗ Do not certify if the driver has:
- Active psychosis;
- Prominent negative symptoms, including substantially compromised judgment, difficulty paying attention, suicidal behavior or ideas, or personality disorder that repeatedly leads to openly inappropriate acts; or
- Treatment side effects that interfere with safe driving.

271

Monitoring/testing: The examiner may order additional tests and/or consult with a mental health specialist, such as a psychiatrist or psychologist, as necessary.

Follow-up: Annual medical exams

Schizophrenia and Related Psychotic Disorders

Schizophrenia is the most severe condition within the spectrum of psychotic disorders. Characteristics of schizophrenia include psychosis (e.g., hearing voices or experiencing delusional thoughts), negative or deficit symptoms (e.g., loss of motivation, apathy, or reduced emotional expression), and compromised cognition, judgment, and/or attention. There is also an increased risk for suicide.

➤ **Individuals with chronic schizophrenia are not considered to be medically qualified for commercial driving.**

Related conditions include:

- Schizophreniform disorder,
- Brief reactive psychosis,
- Schizoaffective disorder, and
- Delusional disorder.

Risks:

A person who is actively psychotic may behave unpredictably in a variety of ways. For example, a person who is hearing voices may receive a command to do something harmful or dangerous, such as self-mutilation. Delusions or hallucinations may lead to violent behavior. Moreover, antipsychotic therapy may cause sedation and motor abnormalities (e.g., muscular rigidity or tremors) and impair coordination, particularly as the medication is being initiated and doses are adjusted.

Waiting period before certification:

- At least 6 months symptom free if brief reactive psychosis or schizophreniform disorder, or

- At least 1 year symptom free if any other psychotic disorder.

Maximum certification: 1 year

Certification recommendations:

 Certify if the driver:
  - Completes the waiting period,

  - Complies with the treatment program,

  - Tolerates treatment without disqualifying side effects, and

  - Is evaluated by a mental health professional who understands the demands of commercial driving.

✗ Do not certify if the driver has:
  - Schizophrenia or active psychosis;

  - Prominent negative symptoms, including substantially compromised judgment, difficulty paying attention, suicidal behavior or ideas, or personality disorder that repeatedly leads to openly inappropriate acts; or

  - Treatment side effects that interfere with safe driving.

NOTE: Chronic schizophrenia is usually a clear-cut condition. Individuals with this condition tend to be severely incapacitated and frequently lack the cognitive skills necessary for steady employment, may have impaired judgment and poor attention, and have a high risk for suicide.

Monitoring/testing: At least every 2 years, the driver with a history of mental illness with psychotic features should be evaluated and cleared for driving by a mental

273

health specialist, such as a psychiatrist or psychologist, who understands the demands of commercial driving.

> The driver should report any manic or severe major depressive episode within 30 days to the driver's employer, medical examiner, or appropriate healthcare professional, and should seek medical care.

Follow-up: Annual medical exams

Antidepressant Therapy

Drivers treated with antidepressant medication are to be evaluated on a case-by-case basis. Some antidepressant drugs significantly interfere with skills performance, but the impact varies widely. With long-term use, many drivers will develop a tolerance to the sedative effects.

First-generation antidepressants have consistently been shown to interfere with safe driving. First-generation antidepressants include tricyclics such as amitriptyline (Elavil) and imipramine (Tofranil).

Second-generation antidepressants have fewer side effects and are generally safe, but can still interfere with safe driving. These include:

- Selective serotonin reuptake inhibitors (SSRIs) such as fluoxetine (Prozac) and sertraline (Zoloft);

- Serotonin and norepinephrine reuptake modulators such as venlafaxine (Effexor); and

- Unicyclic aminoketones such as bupropion (Wellbutrin).

Waiting period before certification: As necessary until the medication is adequate, effective, safe, and stable.

Maximum certification: 1 year

Certification recommendations:

✓ <u>Certify</u> if the underlying condition does not interfere with safe driving, and the effects of the medication do not endanger public safety.

✗ <u>Do not certify</u> if the driver uses a first-generation antidepressant.

NOTE: The FMCSA prefers that drivers using a first-generation tricyclic antidepressant not be certified, stating that "only under exceptional circumstances would continuous use of amitriptyline be acceptable for a commercial driver."

Monitoring/testing: The examiner may order additional tests and/or consult with a mental health specialist, such as a psychiatrist or psychologist, as necessary to evaluate:

- Dose, plasma concentration, and duration of drug therapy; and

- Severity of the underlying mental disorder.

Follow-up: Annual medical exams

Antipsychotic Therapy

Antipsychotic drugs include certain tranquilizers (neuroleptics) that are used to treat schizophrenia, psychotic mood disorders, and some personality disorders, as well as some cases of nausea and chronic pain. Many of the conditions are associated with behaviors and symptoms such as impulsiveness, disturbances in perception and cognition, and an inability to sustain attention. Often the behaviors and symptoms are only partially corrected by drug therapy.

Neuroleptics can cause a variety of side effects that can interfere with driving, such as motor dysfunction that affects coordination and response time, sedation, and visual disturbances, especially at night.

Waiting period before certification: As necessary until the medication is adequate, effective, safe, and stable.

Maximum certification: 1 year

Certification recommendations:

 Certify if:
- The underlying condition does not interfere with safe driving, and

- The effects of medication use while driving do not endanger public safety.

Monitoring/testing: The examiner may order additional tests and/or consult with a mental health specialist, such as a psychiatrist or psychologist, as necessary to evaluate:

- Dose, plasma concentration, and duration of drug therapy; and

- Severity of the underlying mental disorder.

Follow-up: Annual medical exams

Anxiolytic and Sedative Hypnotic Therapy

Anxiolytic (anti-anxiety) drugs used for the treatment of anxiety disorders and to treat insomnia are known as sedative hypnotics, with benzodiazepines being the most common.

Virtually all sedative hypnotics impair skills performance, but the impairment is typically less profound in non-benzodiazepines. However, barbiturates and similar sedative hypnotics cause greater impairment than benzodiazepines. Studies show that the use of benzodiazepines and other sedative hypnotics are probably associated with an increased risk of automobile crashes.

Waiting period before certification: As necessary until the medication is adequate, effective, safe, and stable.

Maximum certification: 2 years

Certification recommendations:

 Certify if the driver uses:
  - A hypnotic, as long as it's short-acting (half-life of less than 5 hours), the lowest effective dose, and used for less than 2 weeks; or

  - A non-sedating anxiolytic.

✕ Do not certify if the driver:
  - Uses a sedating anxiolytic, or

  - Has symptoms or side effects that interfere with safe driving.

Monitoring/testing: The examiner may order additional tests and/or consult with a mental health specialist, such as a psychiatrist or psychologist, as necessary.

Follow-up: At least biennial medical exams (every 2 years)

Electroconvulsive Therapy

Electroconvulsive therapy (ECT) is sometimes used to treat depression. Side effects can include confusion, disorientation, and loss of short-term memory even with low-dose, brief-pulse treatment on one side. Side effects usually resolve rapidly and almost invariably within a few months.

Waiting period before certification: At least 6 months symptom free following a course of ECT.

Certification recommendations:

 Certify if the driver:
- Completes the waiting period;
- Is evaluated by a mental health professional who understands the demands of commercial driving;
- Is not undergoing maintenance ECT; and
- Tolerates treatment without disqualifying side effects.

Monitoring/testing: The examiner may order additional tests and/or consult with a mental health specialist, such as a psychiatrist or psychologist, as necessary.

Follow-up: Annual medical exams

Lithium Therapy

Lithium (Eskalith) is used to treat bipolar and depressive disorders. There is little evidence that lithium interferes with skill performance.

Waiting period before certification: As necessary until the cause is confirmed and treatment is adequate, effective, safe, and stable.

Certification recommendations:

✓ Certify if the driver:
  - Has no side effects,
  - Has lithium levels that are maintained in the therapeutic range, and
  - Has no impairment that interferes with safe driving.

✗ Do not certify if the driver has:
  - A disqualifying underlying condition,
  - Disqualifying symptoms, or
  - Lithium levels that are not in the therapeutic range.

Monitoring/testing: The examiner may order additional tests and/or consult with a mental health specialist, such as a psychiatrist or psychologist, as necessary to evaluate:

- Dose, plasma concentration, and duration of drug therapy; and

- Severity of the underlying mental disorder.

Follow-up: Annual medical exams

VI. *Qualification Standards*

Drug Abuse and Alcoholism

The standard: §391.41(b)(12), (13)

A person is physically qualified to
drive a commercial motor vehicle
(CMV) if that person:

- Does not use a controlled substance
  identified in 21 CFR 1308.11 *Schedule I*, an amphetamine, a narcotic, or any other
  habit-forming drug; or

- Has no current clinical diagnosis of alcoholism.

> **EXCEPTION:** A driver may use a non-Schedule I controlled
> substance or drug if prescribed by a licensed medical
> practitioner who:
>
> - Is familiar with the driver's medical history and assigned
>   duties; and
>
> - Has advised the driver that the prescribed substance or
>   drug will not harm the driver's ability to safely operate a
>   CMV.

Public safety considerations:

There is overwhelming evidence that drug and alcohol
use and/or abuse interferes with driving ability. Although there are separate standards for alcoholism and
other drug problems, many people suffer from both, especially those with antisocial or personality disorders.

Impairment comes from both intoxication and withdrawal. Substance abuse that happens outside of working hours may still cause impairment during
withdrawal. However, when in remission, alcoholism is
not disabling unless temporary or permanent neurological changes have occurred.

Drivers with personality disorders are at especially high risk for drug and/or alcohol dependency, with resulting risks to safety.

Even without abuse, drivers should be aware of the potential harmful effects of mixing drugs (prescription and non-prescription) and alcohol.

Use of medications:

The effects and/or side effects of herbs, supplements, and medications – even those that are taken as legally prescribed – may interfere with safe driving. For example, a driver may experience:

• An altered state of alertness, attention, or temporary confusion; or

• Physical symptoms like low blood pressure, sedation, or increased bleeding that can lead to incapacitation.

In addition, the demands of commercial driving – with irregular and/or extended work/rest/eat patterns – can make it tough to follow the "doctor's orders" for taking medication, and may even increase the need for medication.

Every year, more medications are available without prescription and supervision. Non-prescription medications are not necessarily safe to use while driving

➤ **Drivers are advised to read and understand warning labels on all medications, to store medication properly while on the road, and to consult with a doctor or pharmacist before using new medications or combining medications.**

 Key points:
• The examiner may use drug and/or alcohol abuse screening tests, but the examiner is not authorized to order a "DOT" test as regulated under 49 CFR Part 382.

- A drug or alcohol test is not required as part of the medical certification process.

- Drivers may never use Schedule I drugs, amphetamines, narcotics, methadone, or marijuana.

- Voluntary, ongoing participation in a self-help program to support recovery is not disqualifying.

The exam:

- The driver will be asked for a complete history of medication use, including over-the-counter medications and food and herbal supplements.

- The examiner must evaluate whether the driver has signs of alcoholism, problem drinking, or drug abuse, including tremors or an enlarged liver.

- The examiner may request that the driver's treating physician complete the "391.41 CMV Driver Medication Form" (MCSA-5895), to collect more information about any prescribed medications.

- Drivers may be quizzed about appropriate use and storage of medication while driving, and whether warning labels are being followed.

_____

Alcoholism

Unless there is a current, clinical diagnosis of alcoholism, the medical examiner has discretion to decide if a driver is qualified. If a driver shows signs of alcoholism, he/she may be referred to a specialist for further evaluation.

Alcohol Testing Under Part 382

If the examiner believes *immediate* alcohol testing is
needed, he or she may contact the driver's employer for
information on "reasonable suspicion" drug and alcohol
testing under §382.307. The examiner himself/herself
cannot order a test under Part 382, but could perform a
non-DOT test using a non-DOT form.

Drivers who test positive for alcohol or drugs under
Part 382 are not required to be medically re-examined
or to obtain a new medical examiner's certificate as long
as the driver is seen by a Substance Abuse Professional
(SAP) who evaluates the driver and does not make a
clinical diagnosis of alcoholism.

> **NOTE:** If the SAP determines that alcoholism exists, the driver
> is not qualified to drive a CMV in interstate commerce. The
> ultimate responsibility rests with the motor carrier to ensure the
> driver is medically qualified and to determine whether a new
> medical exam is needed.

Waiting period before certification: As necessary
until the driver has successfully completed counseling
and/or treatment.

Maximum certification: 2 years

STANDARDS

Certification recommendations:

 Certify if the driver with a history of alcoholism:
- Has no lasting disqualifying physical impairment,
- Successfully completed counseling and/or treatment, and
- Has no current disqualifying alcohol-related disorders.

X Do not certify if the driver has:
- A current clinical diagnosis of alcoholism;
- Signs of a current alcoholic illness and/or non-compliance with DOT alcohol guidelines;
- An alcohol-related unstable physical condition, regardless of the time element; or
- Not met return-to-duty requirements.

> **NOTE:** Ongoing, voluntary attendance at self-help groups (e.g., 12-step programs) to aid in recovery is not disqualifying.

Monitoring/testing: The examiner may order additional tests and/or consultation as necessary.

Follow-up: No specific follow up is required.

Drug Abuse

Under 49 CFR Part 382, a CDL driver subject to DOT testing must be removed from safety-sensitive duty when the driver has a verified positive drug test result caused by the unauthorized use of a controlled substance.

The medical examiner himself/herself cannot order a DOT drug test under Part 382, but could perform a non-DOT test using a non-DOT form.

> **NOTE:** When a DOT drug test is required at the same time as a DOT medical exam, a single urine specimen may be used for both. However, the urine to be used for the DOT test must be sealed into the specimen bottles *before* any remaining urine is taken or used for the physical exam (e.g., for glucose testing). See §40.13.

➤ **Drug use or possession is also regulated under §392.4.**

Waiting period before certification: The driver should not be certified for the duration of the prohibited drug use and until a second exam shows the driver is free from the prohibited drug and has completed any recertification requirements.

For a CDL driver to be returned to safety-sensitive duties after failing a DOT drug test, the driver MUST:

• Be evaluated by an SAP,

• Comply with recommended rehabilitation, and

• Have a negative result on a return-to-duty drug test.

Maximum certification: 2 years

Certification recommendations:

 Certify if the driver with a history of drug abuse has:
  • No lasting disqualifying physical conditions; and
  • Proof of successful completion of return-to-duty requirements, if applicable.

✕ Do not certify if the driver uses:
  • Schedule I controlled substances,
  • Amphetamines,
  • Narcotics,
  • Any other habit-forming drug for which the exception guidelines do not apply,

- Methadone (regardless of the reason for the prescription), or
- Marijuana (even if in a state that allows medicinal use).

> **NOTE:** Ongoing voluntary attendance at self-help groups (e.g., 12-step programs) for maintenance of recovery is not disqualifying.

Follow-up: At least biennial exams (every 2 years)

Schedules of Controlled Substances

The federal *Controlled Substances Act* regulates the manufacture, importation, possession, use, and distribution of certain substances. The Act created five schedules or classifications of controlled substances: I, II, III, IV, and V. The drug schedules are based on addiction potential and medical use, and are updated annually.

The Drug Enforcement Administration and the Food and Drug Administration determine which drugs are added to or removed from the various schedules. The schedules can be found under 29 CFR §1308.11 through §1308.15.

According to §391.41(b)(12), a driver's use of Schedule I drugs is medically disqualifying, without exception.

NOTE: Side effects are not part of the DEA schedule rating criteria. Therefore, a substance can have little risk for addiction and abuse but still have side effects that interfere with driving ability.

Schedule I

These drugs have no currently accepted medical use in the United States, cannot legally be prescribed, have a high abuse potential, and are not considered safe, even under medical supervision. These substances include many opiates, opiate derivatives, and hallucinogenic substances. Heroin and marijuana are examples of Schedule I drugs.

- A driver taking "medical" marijuana or any other Schedule I drug cannot be certified under federal standards.

Schedule II

These drugs have accepted medical uses but have a high abuse potential that may lead to severe psychological or physical dependence. Schedule II drugs include opioids, depressants, and amphetamines. The opioids include natural opioids (e.g., morphine) and synthetic opioids (e.g., OxyContin).

- Drivers cannot take methadone, a habit-forming narcotic that appears on Schedule II.

Schedules III - V

These drugs have decreasing potential for abuse. Abuse may lead to moderate or low physical dependence or high psychological dependence.

- Schedule III drugs include tranquilizers.

- Schedule IV drugs include drugs such as chlorhydrol and phenobarbital.

- Schedule V drugs have the lowest potential for abuse and include narcotic compounds or mixtures.

VII. Resolving Conflicts

The Federal Motor Carrier Safety Administration (FMCSA) has procedures in place for resolving situations in which two medical examiners do not agree on the physical qualifications of a driver.

These procedures may be found in §391.47, *Resolution of conflicts of medical evaluation*. The process involves:

1. Seeing an impartial medical specialist in the field in which the medical conflict arose. The specialist should be one agreed to by the motor carrier and the driver. If the specialist cannot resolve the issue, then it must go to the FMCSA.

2. Submission of a written application to the FMCSA by the driver or motor carrier.

NOTE: The driver remains disqualified until the FMCSA makes a decision on the case.

The application must contain or include:

❏ The names and addresses of the driver, motor carrier, and all physicians involved.

❏ Proof that there is a disagreement between the two medical examiners concerning the driver's qualifications.

❏ A copy of the impartial specialist's opinion and report, including results of all tests.

❏ A statement explaining in detail why the decision of the medical specialist is unacceptable.

❏ Proof that the medical specialist was given (prior to his/her determination) the medical history of the driver and an agreed-upon statement of the work the driver performs.

❏ The medical history and statement of work provided to the medical specialist.

❏ All medical records and statements of the physicians who have given opinions on the driver's qualifications.

❏ A description and a copy of all written and documentary evidence on which the applicant relies (see §386.37).

❏ A statement of the driver or motor carrier that he/she intends for the driver to drive in interstate commerce.

These additional documents may be necessary:

IF:	THEN:
the driver refuses to agree on a specialist and the applicant is a motor carrier	the carrier must submit: • A statement of his/her agreement to submit the matter to an impartial specialist, • Proof that he/she has requested the driver to submit to the medical specialist, and • The response, if any, of the driver to that request.
the motor carrier refuses to agree on a specialist	the driver must submit: • An opinion and test results of an impartial specialist, • Proof that he/she has requested the motor carrier to agree to submit the matter to the specialist, and • The response, if any, of the motor carrier to that request.

The applicant must submit three copies of the application and all records.

? Q: What if a motor carrier disagrees with an examiner's certification decision?
A: There are no specific procedures in place for resolving such conflicts. The motor carrier should consult with the examiner, keeping privacy laws in mind.

VIII. Driver Wellness

Note: J. J. Keller & Associates, Inc.® grants permission to purchasers of this Guide to reproduce this chapter for internal use for driver training and educational purposes, provided that J. J. Keller's copyright remains visible on all copies.

Becoming and remaining medically certified takes work. It's up to you – the professional driver – to make the effort to stay healthy and fit so you can continue to drive and perform all the other tasks demanded of your profession.

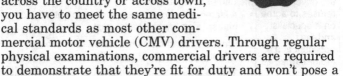

Whether your driving takes you across the country or across town, you have to meet the same medical standards as most other commercial motor vehicle (CMV) drivers. Through regular physical examinations, commercial drivers are required to demonstrate that they're fit for duty and won't pose a danger to themselves or the traveling public.

Fail to live up to those standards and you may find yourself out of a career, at least temporarily.

Highway Safety Begins With You

Each time you turn the key, you are responsible for your own safety, as well as the safety of all the people who share the road with you.

As you know, driving a large truck or bus is not like driving a passenger vehicle. Stopping time and distance, blind spots, and limited maneuverability require drivers to be in top driving performance. It's important to be alert to changes in traffic and to be able to make quick decisions, and the *right* decisions.

Keeping your vehicle in shape also requires *you* to be in shape, to perform pre- and post-trip inspections, loading, unloading, securing cargo, and so on.

Because your good health is important in performing these tasks, the FMCSA mandates standards for a driver's physical well-being. Commercial drivers:

- Must not drive a CMV unless medically qualified;

- Must not drive a CMV if too ill or fatigued to drive safely;

- Must carry proof of medical certification unless such proof is contained in the CDL/CLP driving record;

- Must carry proof of any medical waiver or variance; and

- Must undergo medical exams from DOT-qualified examiners to maintain certification, both on a regular basis as well as following any injury or disease that impairs the ability to drive safety.

NOTE: You and your employer share responsibility for complying with these standards. If you feel your ability to drive or perform other duties has been compromised by an illness, injury, or other medical condition, notify your employer right away and schedule a new DOT medical exam, even if your current medical card is still valid. Though losing your medical certification may be a scary thought, the consequences of a fatal accident would be much more severe!

WELLNESS

Finding an Examiner

If your company does not require you to see a specific medical examiner, you may need to find your own, and you must make sure the examiner is qualified. The easiest (and required) way to do this is to use an examiner who is listed on the National Registry of Certified Medical Examiners. The Registry is searchable online, at:

https://nationalregistry.fmcsa.dot.gov

As long as an examiner is currently listed on the Registry as a qualified examiner, you can use that examiner for your DOT medical exam, no matter where the examiner is located or what the examiner's profession is (e.g., medical doctor, chiropractor, advanced-practice nurse, etc.). You may need to travel to find a qualified examiner if you live in a rural area.

If you are not involved in interstate commerce, then your state may not necessarily require use of the Registry to find a qualified examiner. Check with state enforcement officials for details.

Conversations to Have With Your Doctor

As a CMV driver, you know you're operating a vehicle capable of causing serious harm. You understand that you are equally responsible for the safety of others, and driving a CMV is very different from driving a personal vehicle. It takes skill, knowledge, and a certain level of physical fitness beyond what is required for a passenger car.

As a CMV driver, you need to talk to your doctor about the type of work you do and the physical qualification requirements you must meet to safely operate a CMV. Here are some questions and issues to help in this discussion with your doctor.

1) Tell your doctor what you do, your job responsibilities, and the tasks you perform.

Be sure to include the driving and non-driving tasks, such as the inspections, cargo and baggage distribution, the need to apply chains, etc. By doing this, your doctor will be able to make a better assessment of your health and performance of your job.

2) Ask what effects your injury or illness will have on your job.

What are the direct and indirect impacts on your ability to perform all driving and non-driving tasks safely?

3) Ask about your treatment.

If applicable, ask what you must do or undergo to relieve the symptoms or treat the disease and how the treatment may impact your ability to drive a CMV safely.

4) Ask about alternative treatments.

Ask about equally effective alternate treatments that will not have an adverse impact on safe driving. Would any of these fit your driving requirements better?

5) Ask about the medications your doctor prescribes.

Will the side effects cause sleepiness, fatigue, drowsiness, lack of focus or concentration, or a decreased reaction time? Will the side effects interfere with safe driving?

6) Tell your doctor about the medications you're taking.

Identify prescription and non-prescription drugs, dietary supplements, or herbal remedies, and discuss whether the medications will interact and cause any unsafe side effects. Some medications can interact with one another to cause serious adverse reactions and interfere with the effectiveness of another medication. Don't let your treatment be undone because your medication doesn't work properly!

7) Discuss the extent of treatment and how long you have to take your medication.

8) Ask what you can do to improve your chances for recovery.

Simple changes like losing weight, exercising, avoiding cigarettes, drinking more water, improving your eating

WELLNESS

habits, or getting more sleep can make great improve-
ments in your overall health.

> **Remember:** You're an expert in your work, and your doctor is
> an expert in his or her field. When you put your knowledge
> together, you can come up with a plan designed to meet your
> individual needs, and keep you and those who share the road
> with you, safe.

Special Exceptions

During a DOT medical exam, have you ever been told
that you can't drive a commercial motor vehicle because
you don't meet federal medical standards due to:

- A hearing problem;

- A history of epilepsy, seizures, or similar conditions;
  or

- A missing or impaired limb?

If so, you may be eligible for an exemption from the
medical standards or a special process for becoming certified, which would allow you to operate in interstate
commerce despite the impairment. State-level exemptions often exist for in-state-only drivers as well.

- In the case of the **hearing** and **epilepsy/seizure**
  standards, the FMCSA has exemption applications
  available on its website or by calling (703) 448-3094.

- If you have **monocular vision**, you may be eligible
  for certification if you follow the **alternate vision
  standard** procedures in §391.44.

- If you use **insulin** to control diabetes mellitus, you
  may be eligible for certification if you follow the procedures in §391.46.

- Drivers with missing **limbs** or limb impairments are required to obtain a Skill Performance Evaluation (SPE) certificate. An SPE application is available on the FMCSA's website or by contacting an FMCSA Service Center or calling (202) 366-4001.

> Additional information about federal medical exemptions can be obtained by e-mail to medicalexemptions@dot.gov or fmcsamedical@dot.gov.

NOTE: The FMCSA has no authority to grant a waiver or exemption from a state's in-state requirements.

State exemptions — Individual states can grant exemptions to drivers involved in in-state-only commerce, as long as those drivers do not cross state lines or otherwise get involved in interstate commerce. Vision and diabetes waivers are not uncommon, and states often have "grandfathering" provisions as well. Contact the state's CMV enforcement agency for details.

Medications

Reading a Prescription Label

It's critical to know how medication could make you feel and how it can impact your driving ability and routine. Many people receive a prescription and do not fully understand their medication. When your doctor writes you a prescription, it's very important to ask six basic questions about the medication:

- Why am I taking this medication?

- How much should I take?

- When should I take it?

- How should I take it?

- What should I do if I miss a dose?

- What are the possible side effects?

WELLNESS

VIII. Driver Wellness

You also need to know how the medication will affect your ability to drive. Receiving answers to these questions will help you gain a better understanding of how to read your prescription label(s).

When you get your prescription, remember to verify:

- Your name and address on the prescription label;
- The prescription number and medication name;
- The instructions on taking the medicine; and
- The name of the doctor who wrote the prescription.

Most importantly, know how the medicine could make you feel and how it could affect your daily driving routine. Staying safe is an essential part of managing your health.

Drug Interactions

Medication interactions can occur when you take two or more medications at one time or on the same day. It doesn't matter whether the medication is prescribed, over-the-counter, or herbal.

Interactions can increase or decrease the effectiveness of your medications. When medications interact with chemicals found in the body, in food, or from medical tests, they can cause you to experience serious side effects not normally linked with either drug. These interactions may affect you in many ways, possibly altering the effects of other medications and adversely affecting pre-existing medical conditions.

For instance, blood-pressure medications may cause side effects associated with food intake. If you eat or drink grapefruit products while taking certain blood-pressure medications, you may experience an increased heart rate or blood-pressure changes and/or increased side effects such as facial flushing, headache, or dizziness. Therefore, it's important to inform your healthcare provider of any over-the-counter medications you may be taking.

296

So how can you evaluate your medication interactions to determine if they're major, moderate, or minor?

- **Read labels:** Some medication labels have warnings. These labels may note foods to avoid while taking the medication or the label may say to not take a specific medication in combination with other medications.

- **Speak to your doctor:** In some cases, recommendations from your physician can help manage your interactions.

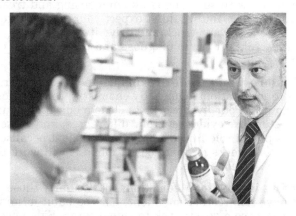

Sharing Medications

Share a cab, share your food, but never share medications. Sharing medications, even over-the-counter medications like aspirin, can be a prescription for disaster.

Side effects and drug interactions: Although it's not uncommon for family and friends to share medications, the medication prescribed for you may cause serious problems for others, with bad side effects such as severe allergic reactions and unhealthy interactions with other medications. In fact, sharing one medication may decrease the effectiveness of another medication. The

WELLNESS

medication you share may work with other prescriptions to double the potency and cause a reaction similar to an overdose. Even herbal and dietary supplements can do this.

Not all symptoms are alike: You may think the symptoms your friend is suffering are the same as yours, but he or she may have a very different medical problem. By sharing your medication, you may be delaying his or her trip to a doctor, and may even contribute to the worsening of a medical condition. Sharing medication with someone is like diagnosing and treating him or her. You wouldn't expect your doctor to get into the cab of your truck and drive it without any training, so don't try to diagnose and treat yourself or your friends.

Unique responses: We are unique and so are our reactions to medications. Our body chemistry, composition, and how fast our liver works to clear medications out of our system are evidence of our differences, and those factors play a role in medication use. So just because a medication works for you doesn't mean it will work the same for someone else.

Sharing is unsafe: Medications, particularly those that have a narcotic component, may be habit-forming and may pose a severe risk to safe driving. Side effects such as drowsiness, dizziness, and confusion have a direct impact on the focus, concentration, and stamina needed for commercial driving. Although you may not have an adverse reaction to the medication, someone else may. Thus, sharing a medication with another driver who may have a different reaction to the medication can cause serious public safety concerns.

It's improper and unsafe to share any prescriptions with other people. Doctor-prescribed medications are strong – even some antibiotics can cause serious reactions – and that's why they have unique numbers for writing prescription orders. Your good intentions may cause dangerous results to health and safety while on or off the road. In addition, sharing a controlled substance such as a narcotic may be illegal.

Wellness

If you spend long hours on the road or on the job, staying healthy and in shape can be tough. But with dedication and persistence, it can be done, often without a huge investment in time or resources. And, staying healthy is critical to obtaining a valid medical card, now and in the future. The following guidance may help.

Eat Right

- Prepare healthy foods at home and take them along. It can be cheaper, quicker, and much healthier than ordering at a restaurant. Thousands of healthy recipes are available – in books, at the library, online, from friends, etc.

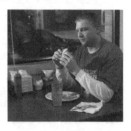

- Eat numerous light meals rather than large, heavy meals that can make you feel fatigued.

- Avoid foods that provide few nutrients and/or are high in fat, salt, and sugars. Look for high-fiber, whole-grain foods, as well as lean proteins and non-fat or low-fat dairy products.

- Cut back on, or eliminate, fried snacks and sugary drinks and choose healthier options like nuts, fruit, oatmeal, yoghurt, water, tea, and granola bars.

- Avoid excessive caffeine.

- Keep a food diary, a log of everything you eat. It can help you take a critical look at your food habits and make healthy changes.

WELLNESS

Exercise

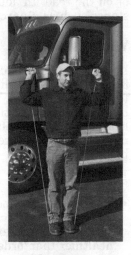

- Physical activity is anything that gets your body moving, and studies say you should do two types of physical activity each week to improve your health and stay strong. Adults need at least:

  - 150 minutes per week of moderate-intensity aerobic activity (e.g., brisk walking), plus muscle-strengthening activities on two or more days a week that work all major muscle groups (legs, hips, back, abdomen, chest, shoulders, and arms); OR

  - 75 minutes per week of vigorous-intensity aerobic activity (e.g., jogging or running), plus muscle-strengthening activities on two or more days a week; OR

  - An equivalent mix of the above.

- If you can't devote long chunks of time to exercise, spread it out! At least 10 minutes at a time is fine. For example, a brisk, 10-minute walk, 3 times a day and 5 days a week, gives you 150 minutes of moderate-intensity activity.

- Walk! Combined with a healthy diet, walking can have a dramatic impact on overall health and can be done without special equipment and at almost any time the opportunity presents itself – maybe when you're sitting at a loading dock, or after lunch, or waiting for passengers or cargo, or when you have some time before or after work. Before you know it, you could be putting in several miles per day.

- If time and budget allows, join a health club and attend regularly.

Avoid Injury

- Stay alert. Watch out for forklifts, machinery, pro-truding nails, spills, and other work hazards.

- When lifting, keep your back straight and avoid twisting. Let your legs do the work.

- Wear gloves and slip-resistant, steel-toed shoes.

- Always have three points of contact with the vehicle when exiting or entering, and never jump from the vehicle or dock.

- Stretch before exerting your muscles, rather than after pulling a muscle.

- Use caution around pressure-loaded equipment like chain binders, steel strapping, tandem and fifth-wheel releases, and trailer doors that have cargo pressing against them.

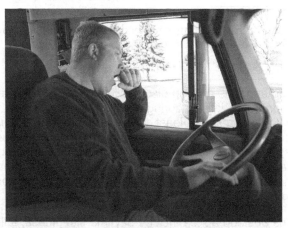

Manage Your Fatigue

Being fatigued impacts your health and could lead to an accident. Major causes of fatigue include lack of sleep and working through or against the body's natural clock, also known as your circadian rhythm. You need to get at least 7 to 8 hours of uninterrupted sleep to be well-rested, and that sleep should come at night whenever possible. A sleep loss of as little as two hours can harm your alertness and performance. Some tips to help get adequate sleep:

- Get plenty of exercise, but no exercise within a couple of hours before bedtime.

- Avoid eating a large meal within three hours before bed. Also, too much liquid may result in a full bladder that keeps you awake.

- Avoid stimulants like caffeine and nicotine before bed, as well as alcohol.

- Stick to a routine, going to bed at night and waking up in the morning at around the same time each day.

- Make sure you have a quiet and comfortable sleep environment.

- Sleep or rest during your body's "low" points, generally 2-6 a.m. and 1-5 p.m.

Sleep Apnea

Sleep apnea is a sleep disorder that causes brief interruptions of breathing during sleep. These pauses in breathing can last at least 10 seconds or more and can occur up to 400 times per night. Sleep apnea is a serious, potentially life-threatening condition that often goes unrecognized and undiagnosed. Studies suggest that almost one-third of commercial drivers may suffer from sleep apnea.

Signs of sleep apnea include daytime sleepiness, falling asleep at inappropriate times, loud snoring, depression, irritability, loss of sex drive, morning headaches, frequent nighttime urination, lack of concentration, and memory impairment. For commercial drivers, these symptoms are dangerous and potentially deadly.

Research indicates that untreated sleep apnea can put you at higher risk for a crash. That's why a diagnosis of moderate to severe sleep apnea can mean the loss of your medical certificate.

Are You at Risk?

Sleep apnea occurs in all age groups and both sexes, but there are certain factors that put you at higher risk. Your doctor may look for these factors during your DOT medical exam and, if necessary, may order additional testing for sleep disorders:

- A family history of sleep apnea;

- Being overweight;

- A large neck size (17 inches or greater for men, 16 inches or greater for women);

- Being age 40 or older;

- Having a small upper airway;

- Having a recessed chin, small jaw, or a large overbite;

- Smoking and alcohol use; and

- Ethnicity.

It Is Treatable

The good news is that sleep apnea is a highly treatable disorder. A continuous positive airway pressure (CPAP) machine is the most effective therapy, requiring patients to wear a nasal mask during sleep. The mask, connected to a pump, gently forces compressed air into the nasal passages at pressures high enough to open the airway from the inside. In addition, people with sleep apnea should lose weight, avoid alcohol prior to bedtime, and avoid sleeping on their backs.

WELLNESS

Other treatments include the wearing of oral devices and surgery to remove enlarged tonsils, adenoids, nasal polyps, or other growths. Deviated nasal septums or unusually formed jaws or soft palates can also be corrected surgically.

Once you have received treatment for sleep apnea and comply with your treatment plan, you can do your job as safely as someone who doesn't have the disorder and can be medically certified.

If you think you might have sleep apnea, discuss the problem with your doctor.

Manage Your Stress

Stress is the body's reaction to the pressure, tension, or the constant change of everyday life, and it can have lasting health effects like high blood pressure, pain, breathing difficulties, digestive problems, insomnia, and fatigue.

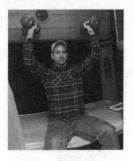

You can manage stress by using one or more of the following stress-reduction techniques:

- Take short breaks and relax.

- Exercise. Even a short walk can help.

- Get plenty of quality rest.

- Start or maintain healthy eating habits.

- Learn and practice stress-relieving techniques such as deep breathing.

- Manage your time – set reasonable priorities and schedules.

IX. Reference

Regulations

Excerpts From 49 CFR §390.5:

Commercial motor vehicle means any self-propelled or towed motor vehicle used on a highway in interstate commerce to transport passengers or property when the vehicle—

1. Has a gross vehicle weight rating or gross combination weight rating, or gross vehicle weight or gross combination weight, of 4,536 kg (10,001 pounds) or more, whichever is greater; or

2. Is designed or used to transport more than 8 passengers (including the driver) for compensation; or

3. Is designed or used to transport more than 15 passengers, including the driver, and is not used to transport passengers for compensation; or

4. Is used in transporting material found by the Secretary of Transportation to be hazardous under 49 U.S.C. 5103 and transported in a quantity requiring placarding under regulations prescribed by the Secretary under 49 CFR, subtitle B, chapter I, subchapter C.

Covered farm vehicle–

1. Means a straight truck or articulated vehicle

   i. Registered in a State with a license plate or other designation issued by the State of registration that allows law enforcement officials to identify it as a farm vehicle;

   ii. Operated by the owner or operator of a farm or ranch, or an employee or family member of a an owner or operator of a farm or ranch;

   iii. Used to transport agricultural commodities, livestock, machinery or supplies to or from a farm or ranch; and

   iv. Not used in for-hire motor carrier operations; however, for-hire motor carrier operations do not include the operation of a vehicle meeting the requirements of paragraphs (1)(i) through (iii) of this definition by a tenant pursuant to a crop share farm lease agreement to transport the landlord's portion of the crops under that agreement.

305

2. Meeting the requirements of paragraphs (1)(i) through (iv) of this definition:

    i. With a gross vehicle weight or gross vehicle weight rating, whichever is greater, of 26,001 pounds or less may utilize the exemptions in §390.39 anywhere in the United States; or

    ii. With a gross vehicle weight or gross vehicle weight rating, whichever is greater, of more than 26,001 pounds may utilize the exemptions in §390.39 anywhere in the State of registration or across State lines within 150 air miles of the farm or ranch with respect to which the vehicle is being operated.

Direct compensation means payment made to the motor carrier by the passengers or a person acting on behalf of the passengers for the transportation services provided, and not included in a total package charge or other assessment for highway transportation services.

Driver means any person who operates any commercial motor vehicle.

Exempt intracity zone means the geographic area of a municipality or the commercial zone of that municipality described in Appendix F to Subchapter B of this Chapter. The term "exempt intracity zone" does not include any municipality or commercial zone in the State of Hawaii. For purposes of §391.62, a driver may be considered to operate a commercial motor vehicle wholly within an exempt intracity zone notwithstanding any common control, management, or arrangement for a continuous carriage or shipment to or from a point without such zone.

Farm vehicle driver means a person who drives only a commercial motor vehicle that is—

a. Controlled and operated by a farmer as a private motor carrier of property;

b. Being used to transport either—

    1. Agricultural products, or

    2. Farm machinery, farm supplies, or both, to or from a farm;

c. Not being used in the operation of a for-hire motor carrier;

d. Not carrying hazardous materials of a type or quantity that requires the commercial motor vehicle to be placarded in accordance with §177.823 of this subtitle; and

e. Being used within 150 air-miles of the farmer's farm.

Farmer means any person who operates a farm or is directly involved in the cultivation of land, crops, or livestock which—

a. Are owned by that person; or

b. Are under the direct control of that person.

Gross combination weight rating (GCWR) is the greater of:

1. A value specified by the manufacturer of the power unit, if such value is displayed on the Federal Motor Vehicle Safety Standard (FMVSS) certification label required by the National Highway Traffic Safety Administration; or

2. The sum of the gross vehicle weight ratings (GVWRs) or the gross vehicle weights (GVWs) of the power unit and the towed unit(s), or any combination thereof, that produces the highest value. Exception: The GCWR of the power unit will not be used to define a commercial motor vehicle when the power unit is not towing another vehicle.

Gross vehicle weight rating (GVWR) means the value specified by the manufacturer as the loaded weight of a single motor vehicle.

Highway means any road, street, or way, whether on public or private property, open to public travel. "Open to public travel" means that the road section is available, except during scheduled periods, extreme weather or emergency conditions, passable by four-wheel standard passenger cars, and open to the general public for use without restrictive gates, prohibitive signs, or regulation other than restrictions based on size, weight, or class of registration. Toll plazas of public toll roads are not considered restrictive gates.

Medical examiner means an individual certified by FMCSA and listed on the National Registry of Certified Medical Examiners in accordance with subpart D of [Part 390].

Medical variance means a driver has received one of the following from FMCSA that allows the driver to be issued a medical certificate:

1. An exemption letter permitting operation of a commercial motor vehicle pursuant to part 381, subpart C, of this chapter or §391.64 of this chapter;

2. A skill performance evaluation certificate permitting operation of a commercial motor vehicle pursuant to §391.49 of this chapter.

49 CFR Part 391, Qualification of Drivers and Longer Combination Vehicle (LCV) Driver Instructors

Subpart E—Physical qualifications and examinations

§391.41 Physical qualifications for drivers.

(a)(1)(i) A person subject to this part must not operate a commercial motor vehicle unless he or she is medically certified as physically qualified to do so, and, except as provided in paragraph (a)(2) of this section, when on-duty has on his or her person the original, or a copy, of a current medical examiner's certificate that he or she is physically qualified to drive a commercial motor vehicle. NOTE: Effective December 29, 1991, and as amended on January 19, 2017, the FMCSA Administrator determined that the Licencia Federal de Conductor issued by the United Mexican States is recognized as proof of medical fitness to drive a CMV. The United States and Canada entered into a Reciprocity Agreement, effective March 30, 1999, recognizing that a Canadian commercial driver's license is proof of medical fitness to drive a CMV. Therefore, Canadian and Mexican CMV drivers are not required to have in their possession a medical examiner's certificate if the driver has been issued, and possesses, a valid commercial driver license issued by the United Mexican States, or a Canadian Province or Territory, and whose license and medical status, including any waiver or exemption, can be electronically verified. Drivers from any of the countries who have received a medical authorization that deviates from the mutually accepted compatible medical standards of the resident country are not qualified to drive a CMV in the other countries. For example, Canadian drivers who do not meet the medical fitness provisions of the Canadian National Safety Code for Motor Carriers but are issued a waiver by one of the Canadian Provinces or Territories, are not qualified to drive a CMV in the United States. In addition, U.S. drivers who received a medical variance from FMCSA are not qualified to drive a CMV in Canada.

(ii) A person who qualifies for the medical examiner's certificate by virtue of having obtained a medical variance from FMCSA, in the form of an exemption letter or a skill performance evaluation certificate, must have on his or her person a copy of the variance documentation when on-duty.

(2) **CDL exception**. (i)(A) Beginning on January 30, 2015 and through June 22, 2025, a driver required to have a commercial driver's license under part 383 of this chapter, and who submitted a current medical examiner's certificate to the State in accordance with 49 CFR 383.71(h) documenting that he or she meets the physical qualification requirements of this part, no longer needs to carry on his or her person the medical examiner's certificate specified at §391.43(h), or a copy, for more than 15 days after the date it was issued as valid proof of medical certification.

(B) On or after June 23, 2025, a driver required to have a commercial driver's license or a commercial learner's permit under 49 CFR part 383, and who has a current medical examiner's certificate documenting that he or she meets the physical qualification requirements of this part, no longer needs to carry on his or her person the medical examiner's certificate specified at §391.43(h).

(ii) Beginning on July 8, 2015, and through June 22, 2025, a driver required to have a commercial learner's permit under part 383 of this chapter, and who submitted a current medical examiner's certificate to the State in accordance with §383.71(h) of this chapter documenting that he or she meets the physical qualification requirements of this part, no longer needs to carry on his or her person the medical examiner's certificate specified at §391.43(h), or a copy for more than 15 days after the date it was issued as valid proof of medical certification.

(iii) A CDL or CLP holder required by §383.71(h) of this chapter to obtain a medical examiner's certificate, who obtained such by virtue of having obtained a medical variance from FMCSA, must continue to have in his or her possession the original or copy of that medical variance documentation at all times when on-duty.

(iv) In the event of a conflict between the medical certification information provided electronically by FMCSA and a paper copy of the medical examiner's certificate, the medical certification information provided electronically by FMCSA shall control.

(3) A person is physically qualified to drive a commercial motor vehicle if:

(i) That person meets the physical qualification standards in paragraph (b) of this section and has complied with the medical examination requirements in §391.43; or

(ii) That person obtained from FMCSA a medical variance from the physical qualification standards in paragraph (b) of this section and has complied with the medical examination requirement in §391.43.

(b) A person is physically qualified to drive a commercial motor vehicle if that person—

(1) Has no loss of a foot, a leg, a hand, or an arm, or has been granted a skill performance evaluation certificate pursuant to §391.49;

(2) Has no impairment of:

(i) A hand or finger which interferes with prehension or power grasping; or

(ii) An arm, foot, or leg which interferes with the ability to perform normal tasks associated with operating a commercial motor vehicle; or any other significant limb defect or limitation which interferes with the ability to perform normal tasks associated with operating a commercial motor vehicle; or has been granted a skill performance evaluation certificate pursuant to §391.49;

(3) Has no established medical history or clinical diagnosis of diabetes mellitus currently treated with insulin for control, unless the person meets the requirements in §391.46;

(4) Has no current clinical diagnosis of myocardial infarction, angina pectoris, coronary insufficiency, thrombosis, or any other cardiovascular disease of a variety known to be accompanied by syncope, dyspnea, collapse, or congestive cardiac failure;

(5) Has no established medical history or clinical diagnosis of a respiratory dysfunction likely to interfere with his/her ability to control and drive a commercial motor vehicle safely;

(6) Has no current clinical diagnosis of high blood pressure likely to interfere with his/her ability to operate a commercial motor vehicle safely;

(7) Has no established medical history or clinical diagnosis of rheumatic, arthritic, orthopedic, muscular, neuromuscular, or vascular disease which interferes with his/her ability to control and operate a commercial motor vehicle safely;

(8) Has no established medical history or clinical diagnosis of epilepsy or any other condition which is likely to cause loss of consciousness or any loss of ability to control a commercial motor vehicle;

(9) Has no mental, nervous, organic, or functional disease or psychiatric disorder likely to interfere with his/her ability to drive a commercial motor vehicle safely;

(10)(i) Has distant visual acuity of at least 20/40 (Snellen) in each eye without corrective lenses or visual acuity separately corrected to 20/40 (Snellen) or better with corrective lenses, distant binocular acuity of at least 20/40 (Snellen) in both eyes with or without corrective lenses, field of vision of at least 70° in the horizontal meridian in each eye, and the ability to recognize the colors of traffic signals and devices showing standard red, green, and amber; or

(ii) Meets the requirements in §391.44, if the person does not satisfy, with the worse eye, either the distant visual acuity standard with corrective lenses or the field of vision standard, or both, in paragraph (b)(10)(i) of this section;

(11) First perceives a forced whispered voice in the better ear at not less than 5 feet with or without the use of a hearing aid or, if tested by use of an audiometric device, does not have an average hearing loss in the better ear greater than 40 decibels at 500 Hz, 1,000 Hz, and 2,000 Hz with or without a hearing aid when the audiometric device is calibrated to American National Standard (formerly ASA Standard) Z24.5—1951;

(12)(i) Does not use any drug or substance identified in 21 CFR 1308.11 Schedule I, an amphetamine, a narcotic, or other habit-forming drug; or

(ii) Does not use any non-Schedule I drug or substance that is identified in the other Schedules in 21 CFR part 1308 except when the use is prescribed by a licensed medical practitioner, as defined in §382.107 of this chapter, who is familiar with the driver's medical history and has advised the driver that the substance will not adversely affect the driver's ability to safely operate a commercial motor vehicle; and

(13) Has no current clinical diagnosis of alcoholism.

§391.43 Medical examination; certificate of physical examination.

(a) Except as provided by paragraph (b) of this section, the medical examination must be performed by a medical examiner listed on the National Registry of Certified Medical Examiners under subpart D of part 390 of this chapter.

(b) Exceptions:

(1) A licensed ophthalmologist or licensed optometrist may perform the part of the medical examination that involves visual acuity, field of vision, and the ability to recognize colors as specified in §391.41(b)(10).

(2) A certified VA medical examiner must only perform medical examinations of veteran operators.

(c) Medical examiners shall:

(1) Be knowledgeable of the specific physical and mental demands associated with operating a commercial motor vehicle and the requirements of this subpart, including the medical advisory criteria prepared by the FMCSA as guidelines to aid the medical examiner in making the qualification determination; and

(2) Be proficient in the use of and use the medical protocols necessary to adequately perform the medical examination required by this section.

(d) Any driver authorized to operate a commercial motor vehicle within an exempt intra city zone pursuant to §391.62 of this part shall furnish the examining medical examiner with a copy of the medical findings that led to the issuance of the first certificate of medical examination which allowed the driver to operate a commercial motor vehicle wholly within an exempt intra city zone.

(e) Any driver operating under a limited exemption authorized by §391.64 shall furnish the medical examiner with a copy of the annual medical findings of the ophthalmologist or optometrist, as required under §391.64. If the medical examiner finds the driver qualified under the limited exemption in §391.64, such fact shall be noted on the Medical Examiner's Certificate.

(f) The medical examination shall be performed, and its results shall be recorded on the Medical Examination Report Form, MCSA-5875, set out in this paragraph (f):

Editor's Note: See Chapter 5 for the medical form that would normally appear here.

(g) Upon completion of the medical examination required by this subpart:

(1) The medical examiner must date and sign the Medical Examination Report and provide his or her full name, office address, and telephone number on the Report.

(2)(i) Before June 23, 2025, if the medical examiner finds that the person examined is physically qualified to operate a commercial motor vehicle in accordance with §391.41(b), he or she must complete a certificate in the form prescribed in paragraph (h) of this section and furnish the original to the person who was examined. The examiner must provide a copy to a prospective or current employing motor carrier who requests it.

(ii) On or after June 23, 2025, if the medical examiner identifies that the person examined will not be operating a commercial motor vehicle that requires a commercial driver's license or a commercial learner's permit and finds that the driver is physically qualified to operate a commercial motor vehicle in accordance with §391.41(b), he or she must complete a certificate in the form prescribed in paragraph (h) of this section and furnish the original to the person who was examined. The examiner must provide a copy to a prospective or current employing motor carrier who requests it.

(3) On or after June 23, 2025, if the medical examiner finds that the person examined is not physically qualified to operate a commercial

motor vehicle in accordance with §391.41(b), he or she must inform the person examined that he or she is not physically qualified, and that this information will be reported to FMCSA. All medical examiner's certificates previously issued to the person are not valid and no longer satisfy the requirements of §391.41(a).

(4) Beginning December 22, 2015, if the medical examiner finds that the determination of whether the person examined is physically qualified to operate a commercial motor vehicle in accordance with §391.41(b) should be delayed to receive additional information or to conduct further examination in order for the medical examiner to make such determination, he or she must inform the person examined that the additional information must be provided or the further examination completed within 45 days, and that the pending status of the examination will be reported to FMCSA.

(5)(i)(A) Once every calendar month, beginning May 21, 2014 and ending on June 22, 2018, the medical examiner must electronically transmit to FMCSA, via a secure Web account on the National Registry, a completed CMV Driver Medical Examination Results Form, MCSA-5850. The Form must include all information specified for each medical examination conducted during the previous month for any driver who is required to be examined by a medical examiner listed on the National Registry of Certified Medical Examiners.

(B) Beginning June 22, 2018 by midnight (local time) of the next calendar day after the medical examiner completes a medical examination for any driver who is required to be examined by a medical examiner listed on the National Registry of Certified Medical Examiners, the medical examiner must electronically transmit to FMCSA, via a secure FMCSA-designated Web site, a completed CMV Driver Medical Examination Results Form, MCSA-5850. The Form must include all information specified for each medical examination conducted for each driver who is required to be examined by a medical examiner listed on the National Registry of Certified Medical Examiners in accordance with the provisions of this subpart E, and should also include information for each driver who is required by a State to be examined by a medical examiner listed on the National Registry of Certified Medical Examiners in accordance with the provisions of this subpart E and any variances from those provisions adopted by such State.

(ii) Beginning on June 22, 2015, if the medical examiner does not perform a medical examination of any driver who is required to be examined by a medical examiner listed on the National Registry of Certified Medical Examiners during any calendar month, the medical examiner must report that fact to FMCSA, via a secure FMCSA-designated Web site, by the close of business on the last day of such month.

(h) The medical examiner's certificate shall be completed in accordance with the following Form MCSA-5876, Medical Examiner's Certificate:

Editor's Note: See Chapter 5 for the medical form that would normally appear here.

(i) Each original (paper or electronic) completed Medical Examination Report and a copy or electronic version of each medical examiner's certificate must be retained on file at the office of the medical examiner for at least 3 years from the date of examination. The medical examiner must make all records and information in these files available to an authorized representative of FMCSA or an authorized Federal, State, or local enforcement agency representative, within 48 hours after the request is made.

§391.44 Physical qualification standards for an individual who does not satisfy, with the worse eye, either the distant visual acuity standard with corrective lenses or the field of vision standard, or both.

(a) **General.** An individual who does not satisfy, with the worse eye, either the distant visual acuity standard with corrective lenses or the field of vision standard, or both, in §391.41(b)(10)(i) is physically qualified to operate a commercial motor vehicle in interstate commerce provided:

(1) The individual meets the other physical qualification standards in §391.41 or has an exemption or skill performance evaluation certificate, if required; and

(2) The individual has the vision evaluation required by paragraph (b) of this section and the medical examination required by paragraph (c) of this section.

(b) **Evaluation by an ophthalmologist or optometrist.** Prior to the examination required by §391.45 or the expiration of a medical examiner's certificate, the individual must be evaluated by a licensed ophthalmologist or licensed optometrist.

(1) During the evaluation of the individual, the ophthalmologist or optometrist must complete the Vision Evaluation Report, Form MCSA-5871.

(2) Upon completion of the Vision Evaluation Report, Form MCSA-5871, the ophthalmologist or optometrist must sign and date the Report and provide the ophthalmologist or optometrist's full name, office address, and telephone number on the Report.

(c) **Examination by a medical examiner.** At least annually, an individual who does not satisfy, with the worse eye, either the distant visual acuity standard with corrective lenses or the field of vision standard, or both, in §391.41(b)(10)(i) must be medically examined and certified by a medical examiner as physically qualified to operate a commercial motor vehicle in accordance with §391.43. The examination must begin not more than 45 days after an ophthalmologist or optometrist signs and dates the Vision Evaluation Report, Form MCSA-5871.

(1) The medical examiner must receive a completed Vision Evaluation Report, Form MCSA-5871, signed and dated by an ophthalmologist or optometrist for each required examination. This Report shall be treated and retained as part of the Medical Examination Report Form, MCSA-5875.

(2) The medical examiner must determine whether the individual meets the physical qualification standards in §391.41 to operate a commercial motor vehicle. In making that determination, the medical examiner must consider the information in the Vision Evaluation Report, Form MCSA-5871, signed by an ophthalmologist or optometrist and, utilizing independent medical judgment, apply the following standards in determining whether the individual may be certified as physically qualified to operate a commercial motor vehicle.

(i) The individual is not physically qualified to operate a commercial motor vehicle if, in the better eye, the distant visual acuity is not at least 20/40 (Snellen), with or without corrective lenses, and the field of vision is not at least 70° in the horizontal meridian.

(ii) The individual is not physically qualified to operate a commercial motor vehicle if the individual is not able to recognize the colors of traffic signals and devices showing standard red, green, and amber.

(iii) The individual is not physically qualified to operate a commercial motor vehicle if the individual's vision deficiency is not stable.

(iv) The individual is not physically qualified to operate a commercial motor vehicle if sufficient time has not passed since the vision deficiency became stable to allow the individual to adapt to and compensate for the change in vision.

(d) **Road test.** (1) Except as provided in paragraphs (d)(3), (4), and (5) of this section, an individual physically qualified under this section for the first time shall not drive a commercial motor vehicle until the individual has successfully completed a road test subsequent to physical qualification and has been issued a certificate of driver's road test in accordance with §391.31. An individual physically qualified under this section for the first time must inform the motor carrier responsible for completing the road test under §391.31(b) that the individual is required by paragraph (d) of this section to have a road test. The motor carrier must conduct the road test in accordance with §391.31(b) thorough (g).

(2) For road tests required by paragraph (d)(1) of this section, the provisions of §391.33 for the equivalent of a road test do not apply. If an individual required to have a road test by paragraph (d)(1) of this section successfully completes the road test and is issued a certificate of driver's road test in accordance with §391.31, then any otherwise applicable provisions of §391.33 will apply thereafter to such individual.

(3) An individual physically qualified under this section for the first time is not required to complete a road test in accordance with §391.31 if the motor carrier responsible for completing the road test under §391.31(b) determines the individual possessed a valid commercial driver's license or non-commercial driver's license to operate, and did operate, a commercial motor vehicle in either intrastate commerce or in interstate commerce excepted by §390.3T(f) of this subchapter or §391.2 from the requirements of this subpart with the vision deficiency for the 3-year period immediately preceding the date of physical qualification under this section for the first time.

(i) The individual must certify in writing to the motor carrier the date the vision deficiency began.

(ii) If the motor carrier determines the individual possessed a valid commercial driver's license or non-commercial driver's license to operate, and did operate, a commercial motor vehicle in either intrastate commerce or in interstate commerce excepted by either §390.3T(f) of this subchapter or §391.2 from the requirements of this subpart with the vision deficiency for the 3-year period immediately preceding the date of physical qualification in accordance with this section for the first time, the motor carrier must—

(A) Prepare a written statement to the effect that the motor carrier determined the individual possessed a valid license and operated a commercial motor vehicle in intrastate or in the specific excepted interstate commerce (as applicable) with the vision deficiency for the 3-year period immediately preceding the date of physical qualification in accordance with this section for the first time and, therefore, is not required by paragraph (d) of this section to complete a road test;

(B) Give the individual a copy of the written statement; and

(C) Retain in the individual's driver qualification file the original of the written statement and the original, or a copy, of the individual's certification regarding the date the vision deficiency began.

(4) An individual physically qualified under this section for the first time is not required to complete a road test in accordance with §391.31 if the individual held on March 22, 2022, a valid exemption from the vision standard in §391.41(b)(10)(i) issued by FMCSA under 49 CFR part 381. Such an individual is not required to inform the motor carrier that the individual is excepted from the requirement in paragraph (d)(1) of this section to have a road test.

(5) An individual physically qualified under this section for the first time is not required to complete a road test in accordance with §391.31 if the individual was medically certified on March 22, 2022, under the provisions of §391.64(b) for drivers who participated in a previous vision waiver study program. Such an individual is not required to inform the motor carrier that the individual is excepted from the requirement in paragraph (d)(1) of this section to have a road test.

§391.45 Persons who must be medically examined and certified.

The following persons must be medically examined and certified in accordance with §391.43 as physically qualified to operate a commercial motor vehicle:

(a) Any person who has not been medically examined and certified as physically qualified to operate a commercial motor vehicle;

(b) Any driver who has not been medically examined and certified as qualified to operate a commercial motor vehicle during the preceding 24 months, unless the driver is required to be examined and certified in accordance with paragraph (c), (d), (e), (f), (g), or (h) of this section;

(c) Any driver authorized to operate a commercial motor vehicle only within an exempt intra-city zone pursuant to §391.62, if such driver has not been medically examined and certified as qualified to drive in such zone during the preceding 12 months;

(d) Any driver authorized to operate a commercial motor vehicle only by operation of the exemption in §391.64, if such driver has not been medically examined and certified as qualified to drive during the preceding 12 months;

(e) Any driver who has diabetes mellitus treated with insulin for control and who has obtained a medical examiner's certificate under the standards in §391.46, if such driver's most recent medical examination and certification as qualified to drive did not occur during the preceding 12 months;

(f) Any driver who does not satisfy, with the worse eye, either the distant visual acuity standard with corrective lenses or the field of vision standard, or both, in §391.41(b)(10)(i) and who has obtained a medical examiner's certificate under the standards in §391.44, if such driver's most recent medical examination and certification as qualified to drive did not occur during the preceding 12 months;

(g) Any driver whose ability to perform his or her normal duties has been impaired by a physical or mental injury or disease; and

(h) On or after June 23, 2025, any person found by a medical examiner not to be physically qualified to operate a commercial motor vehicle under the provisions of paragraph (g)(3) of §391.43.

§391.46 Physical qualification standards for an individual with diabetes mellitus treated with insulin for control.

(a) **Diabetes mellitus treated with insulin**. An individual with diabetes mellitus treated with insulin for control is physically qualified to operate a commercial motor vehicle provided:

(1) The individual otherwise meets the physical qualification standards in §391.41 or has an exemption or skill performance evaluation certificate, if required; and

(2) The individual has the evaluation required by paragraph (b) and the medical examination required by paragraph (c) of this section.

(b) **Evaluation by the treating clinician**. Prior to the examination required by §391.45 or the expiration of a medical examiner's certificate, the individual must be evaluated by his or her "treating clinician." For purposes of this section, "treating clinician" means a healthcare professional who manages, and prescribes insulin for, the treatment of the individual's diabetes mellitus as authorized by the healthcare professional's State licensing authority.

(1) During the evaluation of the individual, the treating clinician must complete the Insulin-Treated Diabetes Mellitus Assessment Form, MCSA-5870.

(2) Upon completion of the Insulin-Treated Diabetes Mellitus Assessment Form, MCSA-5870, the treating clinician must sign and date the Form and provide his or her full name, office address, and telephone number on the Form.

(c) **Medical examiner's examination**. At least annually, but no later than 45 days after the treating clinician signs and dates the Insulin-Treated Diabetes Mellitus Assessment Form, MCSA-5870, an individual with diabetes mellitus treated with insulin for control must be medically examined and certified by a medical examiner as physically qualified in accordance with §391.43 and as free of complications from diabetes mellitus that might impair his or her ability to operate a commercial motor vehicle safely.

(1) The medical examiner must receive a completed Insulin-Treated Diabetes Mellitus Assessment Form, MCSA-5870, signed and dated by the individual's treating clinician for each required examination. This Form shall be treated and retained as part of the Medical Examination Report Form, MCSA-5875.

(2) The medical examiner must determine whether the individual meets the physical qualification standards in §391.41 to operate a commercial motor vehicle. In making that determination, the medical examiner must consider the information in the Insulin-Treated Diabetes Mellitus Assessment Form, MCSA-5870, signed by the treating clinician and, utilizing independent medical judgment, apply the following qualification standards in determining whether the individual with diabetes mellitus treated with insulin for control may be certified as physically qualified to operate a commercial motor vehicle.

(i) The individual is not physically qualified to operate a commercial motor vehicle if he or she is not maintaining a stable insulin regimen and not properly controlling his or her diabetes mellitus.

(ii) The individual is not physically qualified on a permanent basis to operate a commercial motor vehicle if he or she has either severe non-proliferative diabetic retinopathy or proliferative diabetic retinopathy.

(iii) The individual is not physically qualified to operate a commercial motor vehicle up to the maximum 12-month period under §391.45(e) until he or she provides the treating clinician with at least the preceding 3 months of electronic blood glucose self-monitoring records while being treated with insulin that are generated in accordance with paragraph (d) of this section.

(iv) The individual who does not provide the treating clinician with at least the preceding 3 months of electronic blood glucose self-monitoring records while being treated with insulin that are generated in accordance with paragraph (d) of this section is not physically qualified to operate a commercial motor vehicle for more than 3 months. If 3 months of compliant electronic blood glucose self-monitoring records are then provided by the individual to the treating clinician and the treating clinician completes a new Insulin-Treated Diabetes Mellitus Assessment Form, MCSA-5870, the medical examiner may issue a medical examiner's certificate that is valid for up to the maximum 12-month period allowed by §391.45(e) and paragraph (c)(2)(iii) of this section.

(d) **Blood glucose self-monitoring records**. Individuals with diabetes mellitus treated with insulin for control must self-monitor blood glucose in accordance with the specific treatment plan prescribed by the treating clinician. Such individuals must maintain blood glucose records measured with an electronic glucometer that stores all readings, that records the date and time of readings, and from which data can be electronically downloaded. A printout of the electronic blood glucose records or the glucometer must be provided to the treating clinician at the time of any of the evaluations required by this section.

(e) **Severe hypoglycemic episodes**. (1) An individual with diabetes mellitus treated with insulin for control who experiences a severe hypoglycemic episode after being certified as physically qualified to operate a commercial motor vehicle is prohibited from operating a commercial motor vehicle, and must report such occurrence to and be evaluated by a treating clinician as soon as is reasonably practicable. A severe hypoglycemic episode is one that requires the assistance of others, or results in loss of consciousness, seizure, or coma. The prohibition on operating a commercial motor vehicle continues until a treating clinician:

(i) Has determined that the cause of the severe hypoglycemic episode has been addressed;

(ii) Has determined that the individual is maintaining a stable insulin regimen and proper control of his or her diabetes mellitus; and

(iii) Completes a new Insulin-Treated Diabetes Mellitus Assessment Form, MCSA-5870.

(2) The individual must retain the Form and provide it to the medical examiner at the individual's next medical examination.

§391.47 Resolution of conflicts of medical evaluation.

(a) **Applications**. Applications for determination of a driver's medical qualifications under standards in this part will only be accepted if they conform to the requirements of this section.

(b) **Content**. Applications will be accepted for consideration only if the following conditions are met.

(1) The application must contain the name and address of the driver, motor carrier, and all physicians involved in the proceeding.

(2) The applicant must submit proof that there is a disagreement between the physician for the driver and the physician for the motor carrier concerning the driver's qualifications.

(3) The applicant must submit a copy of an opinion and report including results of all tests of an impartial medical specialist in the field in which the medical conflict arose. The specialist should be one agreed to by the motor carrier and the driver.

(i) In cases where the driver refuses to agree on a specialist and the applicant is the motor carrier the applicant must submit a statement of his/her agreement to submit the matter to an impartial medical specialist in the field, proof that he/she has requested the driver to submit to the medical specialist, and the response, if any, of the driver to his/her request.

(ii) In cases where the motor carrier refuses to agree on a medical specialist, the driver must submit an opinion and test results of an impartial medical specialist, proof that he/she has requested the motor carrier to agree to submit the matter to the medical specialist and the response, if any, of the motor carrier to his/her request.

(4) The applicant must include a statement explaining in detail why the decision of the medical specialist identified in paragraph (b)(3) of this section is unacceptable.

(5) The applicant must submit proof that the medical specialist mentioned in paragraph (b)(3) of this section was provided, prior to his/her determination, the medical history of the driver and an agreed-upon statement of the work the driver performs.

(6) The applicant must submit the medical history and statement of work provided to the medical specialist under paragraph (b)(5) of this section.

(7) The applicant must submit all medical records and statements of the physicians who have given opinions on the driver's qualifications.

(8) The applicant must submit a description and a copy of all written and documentary evidence upon which the party making application relies in the form set out in 49 CFR §386.37.

(9) The application must be accompanied by a statement of the driver that he/she intends to drive in interstate commerce not subject to the commercial zone exemption or a statement of the carrier that he/she has used or intends to use the driver for such work.

(10) The applicant must submit three copies of the application and all records.

(c) **Information**. FMCSA (MC-PS) may request further information from the applicant if he/she determines that a decision cannot be made on the evidence submitted. If the applicant fails to submit the information requested, FMCSA may refuse to issue a determination.

(d)(1) **Action**. Upon receiving a satisfactory application FMCSA (MC-PS) shall notify the parties (the driver, motor carrier, or any other interested party) that the application has been accepted and that a determination will be made. A copy of all evidence received shall be attached to the notice.

(2) **Reply**. Any party may submit a reply to the notification within 15 days after service. Such reply must be accompanied by all evidence the party wants FMCSA (MC-PS) to consider in making his/her determination. Evidence submitted should include all medical records and test results upon which the party relies.

(3) **Parties**. A party for the purposes of this section includes the motor carrier and the driver, or anyone else submitting an application.

(e) **Petitions to review, burden of proof**. The driver or motor carrier may petition to review FMCSA's determination. Such petition must be submitted in accordance with §386.13(a) of this chapter. The burden of proof in such a proceeding is on the petitioner.

(f) **Status of driver**. Once an application is submitted to FMCSA (MC-PS), the driver shall be deemed disqualified until such time as FMCSA (MC-PS) makes a determination, or until FMCSA (MC-PS) orders otherwise.

§391.49 Alternative physical qualification standards for the loss or impairment of limbs.

(a) A person who is not physically qualified to drive under §391.41(b)(1) or (b)(2) and who is otherwise qualified to drive a commercial motor vehicle, may drive a commercial motor vehicle if FMCSA has granted a Skill Performance Evaluation (SPE) Certificate to that person.

(b)(1) **Application**. A letter of application for an SPE certificate may be submitted jointly by the person (driver applicant) who seeks an SPE certificate and by the motor carrier that will employ the driver applicant, if the application is accepted.

(2) **Application address.** The application must be addressed to the SPE Certificate Program at the applicable FMCSA service center for the State in which the co-applicant motor carrier's principal place of business is located. The address of each, and the States serviced, are listed in §390.27 of this chapter.

(3) **Exception.** A letter of application for an SPE certificate may be submitted unilaterally by a driver applicant. The application must be addressed to the field service center, FMCSA, for the State in which the driver has legal residence. The driver applicant must comply with all the requirements of paragraph (c) of this section except those in (c)(1)(i) and (iii). The driver applicant shall respond to the requirements of paragraphs (c)(2)(i) to (v) of this section, if the information is known.

(c) A letter of application for an SPE certificate shall contain:
(1) Identification of the applicant(s):
(i) Name and complete address of the motor carrier co-applicant;
(ii) Name and complete address of the driver applicant;
(iii) The U.S. DOT Motor Carrier Identification Number, if known; and
(iv) A description of the driver applicant's limb impairment for which SPE certificate is requested.
(2) Description of the type of operation the driver will be employed to perform:
(i) State(s) in which the driver will operate for the motor carrier co-applicant (if more than 10 States, designate general geographic area only);

(ii) Average period of time the driver will be driving and/or on duty, per day;

(iii) Type of commodities or cargo to be transported;

(iv) Type of driver operation (*i.e.*, sleeper team, relay, owner operator, etc.); and

(v) Number of years experience operating the type of commercial motor vehicle(s) requested in the letter of application and total years of experience operating all types of commercial motor vehicles.

(3) Description of the commercial motor vehicle(s) the driver applicant intends to drive:

(i) Truck, truck tractor, or bus make, model, and year (if known);

(ii) Drive train;

(A) Transmission type (automatic or manual—if manual, designate number of forward speeds);

(B) Auxiliary transmission (if any) and number of forward speeds; and

(C) Rear axle (designate single speed, 2 speed, or 3 speed)

(iii) Type of brake system;

(iv) Steering, manual or power assisted;

(v) Description of type of trailer(s) (i.e., van, flatbed, cargo tank, drop frame, lowboy, or pole);

(vi) Number of semitrailers or full trailers to be towed at one time;

(vii) For commercial motor vehicles designed to transport passengers, indicate the seating capacity of commercial motor vehicle; and

(viii) Description of any modification(s) made to the commercial motor vehicle for the driver applicant; attach photograph(s) where applicable.

(4) Otherwise qualified:

(i) The co-applicant motor carrier must certify that the driver applicant is otherwise qualified under the regulations of this part;

(ii) In the case of a unilateral application, the driver applicant must certify that he/she is otherwise qualified under the regulations of this part.

(5) Signature of applicant(s):

(i) Driver applicant's signature and date signed;

(ii) Motor carrier official's signature (if application has a co-applicant), title, and date signed. Depending upon the motor carrier's organizational structure (corporation, partnership, or proprietorship), the signer of the application shall be an officer, partner, or the proprietor.

(d) The letter of application for an SPE certificate shall be accompanied by:

(1) A copy of the Medical Examination Report Form, MCSA-5875, documenting the results of the medical examination performed pursuant to §391.43;

(2) A copy of the Medical Examiner's Certificate, Form MCSA-5876, completed pursuant to §391.43(h);

(3) A medical evaluation summary completed by either a board qualified or board certified physiatrist (doctor of physical medicine) or orthopedic surgeon. The co-applicant motor carrier or the driver applicant shall provide the physiatrist or orthopedic surgeon with a description of the job-related tasks the driver applicant will be required to perform;

(i) The medical evaluation summary for a driver applicant disqualified under §391.41(b)(1) shall include:

(A) An assessment of the functional capabilities of the driver as they relate to the ability of the driver to perform normal tasks associated with operating a commercial motor vehicle; and

(B) A statement by the examiner that the applicant is capable of demonstrating precision prehension (*e.g.*, manipulating knobs and switches) and power grasp prehension (*e.g.*, holding and maneuvering the steering wheel) with each upper limb separately. This requirement does not apply to an individual who was granted a waiver, absent a prosthetic device, prior to the publication of this amendment.

(ii) The medical evaluation summary for a driver applicant disqualified under §391.41(b)(2) shall include:

(A) An explanation as to how and why the impairment interferes with the ability of the applicant to perform normal tasks associated with operating a commercial motor vehicle;

(B) An assessment and medical opinion of whether the condition will likely remain medically stable over the lifetime of the driver applicant; and

(C) A statement by the examiner that the applicant is capable of demonstrating precision prehension (*e.g.*, manipulating knobs and switches) and power grasp prehension (*e.g.*, holding and maneuvering the steering wheel) with each upper limb separately. This requirement does not apply to an individual who was granted an SPE certificate, absent an orthotic device, prior to the publication of this amendment.

(4) A description of the driver applicant's prosthetic or orthotic device worn, if any;

(5) Road test:

(i) A copy of the driver applicant's road test administered by the motor carrier co-applicant and the certificate issued pursuant to §391.31(b) through (g);

(ii) A unilateral applicant shall be responsible for having a road test administered by a motor carrier or a person who is competent to administer the test and evaluate its results.

(6) Application for employment:

(i) A copy of the driver applicant's application for employment completed pursuant to §391.21; or

(ii) A unilateral applicant shall be responsible for submitting a copy of the last commercial driving position's employment application he/she held. If not previously employed as a commercial driver, so state.

(7) A copy of the driver applicant's SPE certificate of certain physical defects issued by the individual State(s), where applicable; and

(8) A copy of the driver applicant's State Motor Vehicle Driving Record for the past 3 years from each State in which a motor vehicle driver's license or permit has been obtained.

(e) A motor carrier that employs a driver with an SPE certificate agrees to:

(1) File promptly (within 30 days of the involved incident) with the SPE Certificate Program, FMCSA service center, such documents and information as may be required about driving activities, accidents, arrests, license suspensions, revocations, or withdrawals, and convictions which involve the driver applicant. This paragraph (e)(1) applies whether the driver SPE certificate is a unilateral one or has a co-applicant motor carrier;

(i) A motor carrier who is a co-applicant must file the required documents with the SPE Certificate Program, FMCSA service center, for the State in which the carrier's principal place of business is located; or

(ii) A motor carrier who employs a driver who has been issued a unilateral SPE certificate must file the required documents with the SPE

Certificate Program, FMCSA service center, for the State in which the driver has legal residence.

(2) Evaluate the driver with a road test using the trailer the motor carrier intends the driver to transport or, in lieu of, accept a certificate of a trailer road test from another motor carrier if the trailer type(s) is similar, or accept the trailer road test done during the Skill Performance Evaluation if it is a similar trailer type(s) to that of the prospective motor carrier. Job tasks, as stated in paragraph (e)(3) of this section, are not evaluated in the Skill Performance Evaluation;

(3) Evaluate the driver for those nondriving safety related job tasks associated with whatever type of trailer(s) will be used and any other nondriving safety related or job related tasks unique to the operations of the employing motor carrier; and

(4) Use the driver to operate the type of commercial motor vehicle defined in the SPE certificate only when the driver is in compliance with the conditions and limitations of the SPE certificate.

(f) The driver shall supply each employing motor carrier with a copy of the SPE certificate.

(g) FMCSA may require the driver applicant to demonstrate his or her ability to safely operate the commercial motor vehicle(s) the driver intends to drive to an agent of FMCSA. The SPE certificate form will identify the power unit (bus, truck, truck tractor) for which the SPE certificate has been granted. The SPE certificate forms will also identify the trailer type used in the Skill Performance Evaluation; however, the SPE certificate is not limited to that specific trailer type. A driver may use the SPE certificate with other trailer types if a successful trailer road test is completed in accordance with paragraph (e)(2) of this section. Job tasks, as stated in paragraph (e)(3) of this section, are not evaluated during the Skill Performance Evaluation.

(h) FMCSA may deny the application for SPE certificate or may grant it totally or in part and issue the SPE certificate subject to such terms, conditions, and limitations as deemed consistent with the public interest. The SPE certificate is valid for a period not to exceed 2 years from date of issue, and may be renewed 30 days prior to the expiration date.

(i) The SPE certificate renewal application shall be submitted to the SPE Certificate Program, FMCSA service center, for the State in which the driver has legal residence, if the SPE certificate was issued unilaterally. If the SPE certificate has a co-applicant, then the renewal application is submitted to the SPE Certificate Program, FMCSA service center, for the State in which the co-applicant motor carrier's principal place of business is located. The SPE certificate renewal application shall contain the following:

(1) Name and complete address of motor carrier currently employing the applicant;

(2) Name and complete address of the driver;

(3) Effective date of the current SPE certificate;

(4) Expiration date of the current SPE certificate;

(5) Total miles driven under the current SPE certificate;

(6) Number of accidents incurred while driving under the current SPE certificate, including date of the accident(s), number of fatalities, number of injuries, and the estimated dollar amount of property damage;

(7) A current Medical Examination Report Form, MCSA-5875;

(8) A medical evaluation summary pursuant to paragraph (d)(3) of this section, if an unstable medical condition exists. All handicapped conditions classified under §391.41(b)(1) are considered unstable. Refer to paragraph (d)(3)(ii) of this section for the condition under §391.41(b)(2) which may be considered medically stable.

(9) A copy of driver's current State motor vehicle driving record for the period of time the current SPE certificate has been in effect;

(10) Notification of any change in the type of tractor the driver will operate;

(11) Driver's signature and date signed; and

(12) Motor carrier coapplicant's signature and date signed.

(j)(1) Upon granting an SPE certificate, FMCSA will notify the driver applicant and co-applicant motor carrier (if applicable) by letter. The terms, conditions, and limitations of the SPE certificate will be set forth. A motor carrier shall maintain a copy of the SPE certificate in its driver qualification file. A copy of the SPE certificate shall be retained in the motor carrier's file for a period of 3 years after the driver's employment is terminated. The driver applicant shall have the SPE certificate (or a legible copy) in his/her possession whenever on duty.

(2) Upon successful completion of the skill performance evaluation, FMCSA must notify the driver by letter and enclose an SPE certificate substantially in the following form:

Skill Performance Evaluation Certificate

Name of Issuing Agency: _____

Agency Address: _____

Telephone Number: (   ) _____

Issued Under 49 CFR 391.49, subchapter B of the Federal Motor Carrier Safety Regulations

Driver's Name: _____

Effective Date: _____

SSN: _____

DOB: _____

Expiration Date: _____

Address: _____

_____

Driver Disability: _____

Check One: _____ New _____ Renewal

Driver's License: _____
         (State)   (Number)

In accordance with 49 CFR 391.49, subchapter B of the Federal Motor Carrier Safety Regulations (FMCSRs), the driver application for a skill performance evaluation (SPE) certificate is hereby granted authorizing the above-named driver to operate in interstate or foreign commerce under the provisions set forth below. This certificate is granted for the period shown above, not to exceed 2 years, subject to periodic review as may be found necessary. This certificate may be renewed upon submission of a renewal application. Continuation of this certificate is dependent upon strict adherence by the above-named driver to the provisions set forth below and compliance with the FMCSRs. Any failure to comply with provisions herein may be cause for cancellation.

CONDITIONS: As a condition of this certificate, reports of all accidents, arrests, suspensions, revocations, withdrawals of driver licenses or permits, and convictions involving the above-named driver shall be reported in writing to the Issuing Agency by the EMPLOYING MOTOR CARRIER within 30 days after occurrence.

LIMITATIONS:

1. Vehicle Type (power unit):* _____

2. Vehicle modification(s): _____

3. Prosthetic or Orthotic device(s) (Required to be Worn While Driving): _____

4. Additional Provision(s): _____

NOTICE: To all MOTOR CARRIERS employing a driver with an SPE certificate. This certificate is granted for the operation of the *power unit only*. It is the responsibility of the employing motor carrier to evaluate the driver with a road test using the trailer type(s) the motor carrier intends the driver to transport, or in lieu of, accept the trailer road test done during the SPE if it is a similar trailer type(s) to that of the prospective motor carrier. Also, it is the responsibility of the employing motor carrier to evaluate the driver for those non-driving safety-related job tasks associated with the type of trailer(s) utilized, as well as, any other non-driving safety-related or job-related tasks unique to the operations of the employing motor carrier.

The SPE of the above-named driver was given by an SPE Evaluator. It was successfully completed utilizing the above-named power unit and _____ (trailer, if applicable)

The tractor or truck had a _____
transmission.

Please read the *NOTICE* paragraph above.

Name: _____

Signature: _____

Title: _____

Date: _____

(k) FMCSA may revoke an SPE certificate after the person to whom it was issued is given notice of the proposed revocation and has been allowed a reasonable opportunity to appeal.

(l) Falsifying information in the letter of application, the renewal application, or falsifying information required by this section by either the applicant or motor carrier is prohibited.

APPENDIX A TO PART 391—MEDICAL ADVISORY CRITERIA

I. Introduction

This appendix contains the Agency's guidelines in the form of Medical Advisory Criteria to help medical examiners assess a driver's physical qualification. These guidelines are strictly advisory and were established after consultation with physicians, States, and industry representatives, and, in some areas, after consideration of recommendations from the Federal Motor Carrier Safety Administration's Medical Review Board and Medical Expert Panels.

II. Interpretation of Medical Standards

Since the issuance of the regulations for physical qualifications of commercial motor vehicle drivers, the Federal Motor Carrier Safety Administration has published recommendations called Advisory Criteria to help medical examiners in determining whether a driver meets the physical qualifications for commercial driving. These recommendations have been condensed to provide information to medical examiners that is directly relevant to the physical examination and is not already included in the Medical Examination Report Form.

A. Loss of Limb: §391.41(b)(1)

A person is physically qualified to drive a commercial motor vehicle if that person: Has no loss of a foot, leg, hand or an arm, or has been granted a Skills Performance Evaluation certificate pursuant to §391.49.

B. Limb Impairment: §391.41(b)(2)

1. A person is physically qualified to drive a commercial motor vehicle if that person: Has no impairment of:

(i) A hand or finger which interferes with prehension or power grasping; or

(ii) An arm, foot, or leg which interferes with the ability to perform normal tasks associated with operating a commercial motor vehicle; or

(iii) Any other significant limb defect or limitation which interferes with the ability to perform normal tasks associated with operating a commercial motor vehicle; or

(iv) Has been granted a Skills Performance Evaluation certificate pursuant to §391.49.

2. A person who suffers loss of a foot, leg, hand or arm or whose limb impairment in any way interferes with the safe performance of normal tasks associated with operating a commercial motor vehicle is subject to the Skills Performance Evaluation Certificate Program pursuant to §391.49, assuming the person is otherwise qualified.

3. With the advancement of technology, medical aids and equipment modifications have been developed to compensate for certain disabilities. The Skills Performance Evaluation Certificate Program (formerly the Limb Waiver Program) was designed to allow persons with the loss of a foot or limb or with functional impairment to qualify under the Federal Motor Carrier Safety Regulations by use of prosthetic devices or equipment modifications which enable them to safely operate a commercial motor vehicle. Since there are no medical aids equivalent to the original body or limb, certain risks are still present, and thus restrictions may be included on individual Skills Performance Evaluation certificates when a State Director for the Federal Motor Carrier Safety Administration determines they are necessary to be consistent with safety and public interest.

4. If the driver is found otherwise medically qualified (§391.41(b)(3) through (13)), the medical examiner must check on the Medical Examiner's Certificate that the driver is qualified only if accompanied by a Skills Performance Evaluation certificate. The driver and the employing motor carrier are subject to appropriate penalty if the driver operates a motor vehicle in interstate or foreign commerce without a current Skill Performance Evaluation certificate for his/her physical disability.

C. [Reserved]

IX. Reference

D. Cardiovascular Condition: §391.41(b)(4)

1. A person is physically qualified to drive a commercial motor vehicle if that person: Has no current clinical diagnosis of myocardial infarction, angina pectoris, coronary insufficiency, thrombosis or any other cardiovascular disease of a variety known to be accompanied by syncope, dyspnea, collapse or congestive cardiac failure.

2. The term "has no current clinical diagnosis of" is specifically designed to encompass: "a clinical diagnosis of" a current cardiovascular condition, or a cardiovascular condition which has not fully stabilized regardless of the time limit. The term "known to be accompanied by" is designed to include a clinical diagnosis of a cardiovascular disease which is accompanied by symptoms of syncope, dyspnea, collapse or congestive cardiac failure; and/or which is s likely to cause syncope, dyspnea, collapse or congestive cardiac failure.

3. It is the intent of the Federal Motor Carrier Safety Regulations to render unqualified, a driver who has a current cardiovascular disease which is accompanied by and/or likely to cause symptoms of syncope, dyspnea, collapse, or congestive cardiac failure. However, the subjective decision of whether the nature and severity of an individual's condition will likely cause symptoms of cardiovascular insufficiency is on an individual basis and qualification rests with the medical examiner and the motor carrier. In those cases where there is an occurrence of cardiovascular insufficiency (myocardial infarction, thrombosis, etc.), it is suggested before a driver is certified that he or she have a normal resting and stress electrocardiogram, no residual complications and no physical limitations, and is taking no medication likely to interfere with safe driving.

4. Coronary artery bypass surgery and pacemaker implantation are remedial procedures and thus, not medically disqualifying. Implantable cardioverter defibrillators are disqualifying due to risk of syncope. Coumadin is a medical treatment which can improve the health and safety of the driver and should not, by its use, medically disqualify the commercial motor vehicle driver. The emphasis should be on the underlying medical condition(s) which require treatment and the general health of the driver. The Federal Motor Carrier Safety Administration should be contacted at (202) 366-4001 for additional recommendations regarding the physical qualification of drivers on coumadin.

E. Respiratory Dysfunction: §391.41(b)(5)

1. A person is physically qualified to drive a commercial motor vehicle if that person: Has no established medical history or clinical diagnosis of a respiratory dysfunction likely to interfere with ability to control and drive a commercial motor vehicle safely.

2. Since a driver must be alert at all times, any change in his or her mental state is in direct conflict with highway safety. Even the slightest impairment in respiratory function under emergency conditions (when greater oxygen supply is necessary for performance) may be detrimental to safe driving.

3. There are many conditions that interfere with oxygen exchange and may result in incapacitation, including emphysema, chronic asthma, carcinoma, tuberculosis, chronic bronchitis and sleep apnea. If the medical examiner detects a respiratory dysfunction, that in any way is likely to interfere with the driver's ability to safely control and drive a commercial motor vehicle, the driver must be referred to a specialist for further evaluation and therapy. Anticoagulation therapy for deep vein thrombosis and/or pulmonary thromboembolism is not medically disqualifying once optimum dose is achieved, provided lower extremity venous examinations remain normal and the treating physician gives a favorable recommendation.

326

F. Hypertension: §391.41(b)(6)

1. A person is physically qualified to drive a commercial motor vehicle if that person: Has no current clinical diagnosis of high blood pressure likely to interfere with ability to operate a commercial motor vehicle safely.

2. Hypertension alone is unlikely to cause sudden collapse; however, the likelihood increases when target organ damage, particularly cerebral vascular disease, is present. This regulatory criteria is based on the Federal Motor Carrier Safety Administration's Cardiovascular Advisory Guidelines for the Examination of commercial motor vehicle Drivers, which used the Sixth Report of the Joint National Committee on Detection, Evaluation, and Treatment of High Blood Pressure (1997).

3. Stage 1 hypertension corresponds to a systolic blood pressure of 140-159 mmHg and/or a diastolic blood pressure of 90-99 mmHg. The driver with a blood pressure in this range is at low risk for hypertension-related acute incapacitation and may be medically certified to drive for a one-year period. Certification examinations should be done annually thereafter and should be at or less than 140/90. If less than 160/100, certification may be extended one time for 3 months.

4. A blood pressure of 160-179 systolic and/or 100-109 diastolic is considered Stage 2 hypertension, and the driver is not necessarily unqualified during evaluation and institution of treatment. The driver is given a one-time certification of three months to reduce his or her blood pressure to less than or equal to 140/90. A blood pressure in this range is an absolute indication for anti-hypertensive drug therapy. Provided treatment is well tolerated and the driver demonstrates a blood pressure value of 140/90 or less, he or she may be certified for one year from date of the initial exam. The driver is certified annually thereafter.

5. A blood pressure at or greater than 180 (systolic) and 110 (diastolic) is considered Stage 3, high risk for an acute blood pressure-related event. The driver may not be qualified, even temporarily, until reduced to 140/90 or less and treatment is well tolerated. The driver may be certified for 6 months and biannually (every 6 months) thereafter if at recheck blood pressure is 140/90 or less.

6. Annual recertification is recommended if the medical examiner does not know the severity of hypertension prior to treatment. An elevated blood pressure finding should be confirmed by at least two subsequent measurements on different days.

7. Treatment includes nonpharmacologic and pharmacologic modalities as well as counseling to reduce other risk factors. Most antihypertensive medications also have side effects, the importance of which must be judged on an individual basis. Individuals must be alerted to the hazards of these medications while driving. Side effects of somnolence or syncope are particularly undesirable in commercial motor vehicle drivers.

8. Secondary hypertension is based on the above stages. Evaluation is warranted if patient is persistently hypertensive on maximal or near-maximal doses of 2-3 pharmacologic agents. Some causes of secondary hypertension may be amenable to surgical intervention or specific pharmacologic disease.

G. Rheumatic, Arthritic, Orthopedic, Muscular, Neuromuscular or Vascular Disease: §391.41(b)(7)

1. A person is physically qualified to drive a commercial motor vehicle if that person: Has no established medical history or clinical diagnosis of rheumatic, arthritic, orthopedic, muscular, neuromuscular or vascular disease which interferes with the ability to control and operate a commercial motor vehicle safely.

327

IX. Reference

2. Certain diseases are known to have acute episodes of transient muscle weakness, poor muscular coordination (ataxia), abnormal sensations (paresthesia), decreased muscular tone (hypotonia), visual disturbances and pain which may be suddenly incapacitating. With each recurring episode, these symptoms may become more pronounced and remain for longer periods of time. Other diseases have more insidious onsets and display symptoms of muscle wasting (atrophy), swelling and paresthesia which may not suddenly incapacitate a person but may restrict his/her movements and eventually interfere with the ability to safely operate a motor vehicle. In many instances these diseases are degenerative in nature or may result in deterioration of the involved area.

3. Once the individual has been diagnosed as having a rheumatic, arthritic, orthopedic, muscular, neuromuscular or vascular disease, then he/she has an established history of that disease. The physician, when examining an individual, should consider the following: The nature and severity of the individual's condition (such as sensory loss or loss of strength); the degree of limitation present (such as range of motion); the likelihood of progressive limitation (not always present initially but may manifest itself over time); and the likelihood of sudden incapacitation. If severe functional impairment exists, the driver does not qualify. In cases where more frequent monitoring is required, a certificate for a shorter period of time may be issued.

H. Epilepsy: §391.41(b)(8)

1. A person is physically qualified to drive a commercial motor vehicle if that person: Has no established medical history or clinical diagnosis of epilepsy or any other condition which is likely to cause loss of consciousness or any loss of ability to control a motor vehicle.

2. Epilepsy is a chronic functional disease characterized by seizures or episodes that occur without warning, resulting in loss of voluntary control which may lead to loss of consciousness and/or seizures. Therefore, the following drivers cannot be qualified:

(i) A driver who has a medical history of epilepsy;

(ii) A driver who has a current clinical diagnosis of epilepsy; or

(ii) A driver who is taking antiseizure medication.

3. If an individual has had a sudden episode of a nonepileptic seizure or loss of consciousness of unknown cause which did not require antiseizure medication, the decision as to whether that person's condition will likely cause loss of consciousness or loss of ability to control a motor vehicle is made on an individual basis by the medical examiner in consultation with the treating physician. Before certification is considered, it is suggested that a 6 month waiting period elapse from the time of the episode. Following the waiting period, it is suggested that the individual have a complete neurological examination. If the results of the examination are negative and antiseizure medication is not required, then the driver may be qualified.

4. In those individual cases where a driver has a seizure or an episode of loss of consciousness that resulted from a known medical condition (*e.g.*, drug reaction, high temperature, acute infectious disease, dehydration or acute metabolic disturbance), certification should be deferred until the driver has fully recovered from that condition and has no existing residual complications, and not taking antiseizure medication.

5. Drivers with a history of epilepsy/seizures off antiseizure medication and seizure-free for 10 years may be qualified to drive a commercial motor vehicle in interstate commerce. Interstate drivers with a history of a single unprovoked seizure may be

qualified to drive a commercial motor vehicle in interstate commerce if seizure-free and off antiseizure medication for a 5-year period or more.

I. Mental Disorders: §391.41(b)(9)

1. A person is physically qualified to drive a commercial motor vehicle if that person: Has no mental, nervous, organic or functional disease or psychiatric disorder likely to interfere with ability to drive a motor vehicle safely.

2. Emotional or adjustment problems contribute directly to an individual's level of memory, reasoning, attention, and judgment. These problems often underlie physical disorders. A variety of functional disorders can cause drowsiness, dizziness, confusion, weakness or paralysis that may lead to incoordination, inattention, loss of functional control and susceptibility to accidents while driving. Physical fatigue, headache, impaired coordination, recurring physical ailments and chronic "nagging" pain may be present to such a degree that certification for commercial driving is inadvisable. Somatic and psychosomatic complaints should be thoroughly examined when determining an individual's overall fitness to drive. Disorders of a periodically incapacitating nature, even in the early stages of development, may warrant disqualification.

3. Many bus and truck drivers have documented that "nervous trouble" related to neurotic, personality, or emotional or adjustment problems is responsible for a significant fraction of their preventable accidents. The degree to which an individual is able to appreciate, evaluate and adequately respond to environmental strain and emotional stress is critical when assessing an individual's mental alertness and flexibility to cope with the stresses of commercial motor vehicle driving.

4. When examining the driver, it should be kept in mind that individuals who live under chronic emotional upsets may have deeply ingrained maladaptive or erratic behavior patterns. Excessively antagonistic, instinctive, impulsive, openly aggressive, paranoid or severely depressed behavior greatly interfere with the driver's ability to drive safely. Those individuals who are highly susceptible to frequent states of emotional instability (schizophrenia, affective psychoses, paranoia, anxiety or depressive neuroses) may warrant disqualification. Careful consideration should be given to the side effects and interactions of medications in the overall qualification determination.

J. [Reserved]

K. Hearing: §391.41(b)(11)

1. A person is physically qualified to drive a commercial motor vehicle if that person: First perceives a forced whispered voice in the better ear at not less than 5 feet with or without the use of a hearing aid, or, if tested by use of an audiometric device, does not have an average hearing loss in the better ear greater than 40 decibels at 500 Hz, 1,000 Hz, and 2,000 Hz with or without a hearing aid when the audiometric device is calibrated to American National Standard (formerly ADA Standard) Z24.5-1951.

2. Since the prescribed standard under the Federal Motor Carrier Safety Regulations is from the American National Standards Institute, formerly the American Standards Association, it may be necessary to convert the audiometric results from the International Organization for Standardization standard to the American National Standards Institute standard. Instructions are included on the Medical Examination Report Form.

3. If an individual meets the criteria by using a hearing aid, the driver must wear that hearing aid and have it in operation at all times while driving. Also, the driver must be in possession of a spare power source for the hearing aid.

4. For the whispered voice test, the individual should be stationed at least 5 feet from the medical examiner with the ear being tested turned toward the medical examiner. The other ear is covered. Using the breath which remains after a normal expiration, the medical examiner whispers words or random numbers such as 66, 18, 3, etc. The medical examiner should not use only sibilants (s sounding materials). The opposite ear should be tested in the same manner.

5. If the individual fails the whispered voice test, the audiometric test should be administered. If an individual meets the criteria by the use of a hearing aid, the following statement must appear on the Medical Examiner's Certificate "Qualified only when wearing a hearing aid."

L. Drug Use: §391.41(b)(12)

1. A person is physically qualified to drive a commercial motor vehicle if that person does not use any drug or substance identified in 21 CFR 1308.11, an amphetamine, a narcotic, or other habit-forming drug. A driver may use a non-Schedule I drug or substance that is identified in the other Schedules in 21 CFR part 1308 if the substance or drug is prescribed by a licensed medical practitioner who:

(i) Is familiar with the driver's medical history, and assigned duties; and

(ii) Has advised the driver that the prescribed substance or drug will not adversely affect the driver's ability to safely operate a commercial motor vehicle.

2. This exception does not apply to methadone. The intent of the medical certification process is to medically evaluate a driver to ensure that the driver has no medical condition which interferes with the safe performance of driving tasks on a public road. If a driver uses an amphetamine, a narcotic or any other habit-forming drug, it may be cause for the driver to be found medically unqualified. If a driver uses a Schedule I drug or substance, it will be cause for the driver to be found medically unqualified. Motor carriers are encouraged to obtain a practitioner's written statement about the effects on transportation safety of the use of a particular drug.

3. A test for controlled substances is not required as part of this biennial certification process. The Federal Motor Carrier Safety Administration or the driver's employer should be contacted directly for information on controlled substances and alcohol testing under Part 382 of the FMCSRs.

4. The term "uses" is designed to encompass instances of prohibited drug use determined by a physician through established medical means. This may or may not involve body fluid testing. If body fluid testing takes place, positive test results should be confirmed by a second test of greater specificity. The term "habit-forming" is intended to include any drug or medication generally recognized as capable of becoming habitual, and which may impair the user's ability to operate a commercial motor vehicle safely.

5. The driver is medically unqualified for the duration of the prohibited drug(s) use and until a second examination shows the driver is free from the prohibited drug(s) use. Recertification may involve a substance abuse evaluation, the successful completion of a drug rehabilitation program, and a negative drug test result. Additionally, given that the certification period is normally two years, the medical examiner has the option to certify for a period of less than 2 years if this medical examiner determines more frequent monitoring is required.

M. Alcoholism: §391.41(b)(13)

1. A person is physically qualified to drive a commercial motor vehicle if that person: Has no current clinical diagnosis of alcoholism.

2. The term "current clinical diagnosis of" is specifically designed to encompass a current alcoholic illness or those instances where the individual's physical condition has not fully stabilized, regardless of the time element. If an individual shows signs of having an alcohol-use problem, he or she should be referred to a specialist. After counseling and/or treatment, he or she may be considered for certification.

FMCSA Interpretations

§391.41 Physical qualifications for drivers

Question 1: Who is responsible for ensuring that medical certifications meet the requirements?

Guidance: Medical certification determinations are the responsibility of the medical examiner. The motor carrier has the responsibility to ensure that the medical examiner is informed of the minimum medical requirements and the characteristics of the work to be performed. The motor carrier is also responsible for ensuring that only medically qualified drivers are operating CMVs in interstate commerce.

Question 2: Do the physical qualification requirements of the FMCSRs infringe upon a person's religious beliefs if such beliefs prohibit being examined by a licensed doctor of medicine or osteopathy?

Guidance: No. To determine whether a governmental regulation infringes on a person's right to freely practice his religion, the interest served by the regulation must be balanced against the degree to which a person's rights are adversely affected. *Biklen v. Board of Education*, 333 F. Supp. 902 (N.D.N.Y. 1971) aff'd 406 U.S. 951 (1972).

If there is an important objective being promoted by the requirement and the restriction on religious freedom is reasonably adapted to achieving that objective, the requirement should be upheld. *Burgin v. Henderson*, 536 F.2d 501 (2d. Cir. 1976). Based on the tests developed by the courts and the important objective served, the regulation meets Constitutional standards. It does not deny a driver his First Amendment rights.

Question 3: What are the physical qualification requirements for operating a CMV in interstate commerce?

Guidance: The physical qualification regulations for drivers in interstate commerce are found at §391.41. Instructions to medical examiners performing physical qualification examinations of these drivers are found at §391.43.

IX. Reference

The qualification standards cover 13 areas, which directly relate to the driving function. All but two of the standards require a judgment by the medical examiner. A person's qualification to drive is determined by a medical examiner who is knowledgeable about the driver's functions and whether the driver's physical condition is adequate to enable the driver to operate the vehicle safely. In the case of hearing and epilepsy, the current standards are absolute, providing no discretion to the medical examiner. However, drivers who do not meet the current requirements may apply for an exemption as provided by 49 CFR part 381.

Question 4: Is a driver who is taking prescription methadone qualified to drive a CMV in interstate commerce?

Guidance: Methadone is a habit-forming narcotic which can produce drug dependence and is not an allowable drug for operators of CMVs.

Question 5: May the medical examiner restrict a driver's duties?

Guidance: No. The only conditions a medical examiner may impose upon a driver otherwise qualified involve the use of corrective lenses or hearing aids, securement of a waiver or limitation of driving to exempt intracity zones (see §391.43(g)). A medical examiner who believes a driver has a condition not specified in §391.41 that would affect his ability to operate a CMV safely should refuse to sign the examiner's certificate.

Question 6: If an interstate driver tests positive for alcohol or controlled substances under part 382, must the driver be medically re-examined and obtain a new medical examiner's certificate to drive again?

Guidance: The driver is not required to be medically re-examined or to obtain a new medical examiner's certificate *provided* the driver is seen by an SAP who evaluates the driver, does not make a clinical diagnosis of alcoholism, and provides the driver with documentation allowing the driver to return to work. However, if the SAP determines that alcoholism exists, the driver is not qualified to drive a CMV in interstate commerce. The ultimate responsibility rests with the motor carrier to ensure the driver is medically qualified and to determine whether a new medical examination should be completed.

Question 7: Are drivers prohibited from using CB radios and earphones?

Guidance: No. CB radios and earphones are not prohibited under the regulations, as long as they do not distract the driver and the driver is capable of complying with §391.41(b)(11).

Question 8: Is the use of coumadin, an anticoagulant, an automatic disqualification for drivers operating CMVs in interstate commerce?

Guidance: No. Although the FHWA 1987 "Conference on Cardiac Disorders and Commercial Drivers" recommended that drivers who are taking anticoagulants not be allowed to drive, the agency has not adopted a rule to that effect. The medical examiner and treating specialist may, but are not required to, accept the Conference recommendations. Therefore, the use of coumadin is not an automatic disqualification, but a factor to be considered in determining the driver's physical qualification status.

§391.43 Medical examination; certificate of physical examination

Question 1: May a motor carrier, for the purposes of §391.41, or a State driver licensing agency, for the purposes of §383.71, accept the results of a medical examination performed by a foreign medical examiner?

Guidance: Yes. Foreign drivers operating in the U.S. with a driver's license recognized as equivalent to the CDL may be medically certified in accordance with the requirements of part 391, subpart E, by a medical examiner in the driver's home country who is licensed, certified, and/or registered to perform physical examinations in that country. *However*, U.S. drivers operating in interstate commerce within the U.S. must be medically certified in accordance with part 391, subpart E, by a medical examiner licensed, certified, and/or registered to perform physical examinations in the U.S.

Question 2: May a urine sample collected for purposes of performing a subpart H test be used to test for diabetes as part of a driver's FHWA-required physical examination?

Guidance: In general, no. However, the DOT has recognized an exception to this general policy whereby, after 60 milliliters of urine have been set aside for subpart H testing, any remaining portion of the sample may be used for other nondrug testing, but only if such other nondrug testing is required by the FHWA (under part 391, subpart E) such as testing for glucose and protein levels.

Question 3: Is a chest x-ray required under the minimum medical requirements of the FMCSRs?

Guidance: No, but a medical examiner may take an x-ray if appropriate.

Question 4: Does §391.43 of the FMCSRs require that physical examinations of applicants for employment be conducted by medical examiners employed by or designated by the carrier?

Guidance: No.

Question 5: Does a medical certificate displaying a facsimile of a medical examiner's signature meet the "signature of examining health care professional" requirement?

Guidance: Yes.

Question 6: The driver's medical exam is part of the Mexican Licencia Federal. If a roadside inspection reveals that a Mexico-based driver has not had the medical portion of the Licencia Federal re-validated, is the driver considered to be without a valid medical certificate or without a valid license?

Guidance: The Mexican Licencia Federal is issued for a period of 10 years but must be re-validated every 2 years. A condition of re-validation is that the driver must pass a new physical examination. The dates for each re-validation are on the Licencia Federal and must be stamped at the completion of each physical. This constitutes documentation that the driver is medically qualified. Therefore, if the Licencia Federal is not re-validated every 2 years as specified by Mexican law, the driver's license is considered invalid.

*Question 7: If a motor carrier sends a potential interstate driver to a medical examiner to have both a pre-employment medical examination and a pre-employment controlled substances test performed, how must the medical examiner conduct the medical examination including the certification the driver meets the physical qualifications of §391.41(b)?

Guidance: The medical examiner must complete the physical examination first without collecting the Part 382 controlled substances urine specimen. If the potential driver meets the requirements of Part 391, Subpart E [especially §391.41(b)] and the medical examiner chooses to certify the potential driver as qualified to operate commercial motor vehicles (CMV) in interstate commerce, the medical examiner may prepare the medical examiner's certificate.

After the medical examiner has completed the medical examiner's certificate and provided a copy to the potential driver and to the motor carrier who will use the potential driver's services, the medical examiner may collect the specimen for the 49 CFR Part 382 pre-employment controlled substances test. The motor carrier is held fully responsible for ensuring the potential driver is not used to operate CMVs until the carrier receives a verified negative controlled substances test result from the medical review officer. A Department of Transportation pre-employment controlled substances test is not a medical examination test.

*Editor's Note: This interpretation was issued after the interpretations were published in the *Federal Register* in April 1997.

§391.45 Persons who must be medically examined and certified

Question 1: Is it intended that the words "person" and "driver" be used interchangeably in §391.45?

Guidance: Yes.

Question 2: Do the FMCSRs require applicants, possessing a current medical certificate, to undergo a new physical examination as a condition of employment?

Guidance: No. However, if a motor carrier accepts such a currently valid certificate from a driver subject to part 382, the driver is subject to additional controlled substance testing requirements unless otherwise excepted in subpart H.

334

Question 3: Must a driver who is returning from an illness or injury undergo a medical examination even if his current medical certificate has not expired?

Guidance: The FMCSRs do not require an examination in this case unless the injury or illness has impaired the driver's ability to perform his/her normal duties. However, the motor carrier may require a driver returning from any illness or injury to take a physical examination. But, in either case, the motor carrier has the obligation to determine if an injury or illness renders the driver medically unqualified.

§391.47 Resolution of conflicts of medical evaluation

Question 1: Does the FHWA issue formal medical decisions as to the physical qualifications of drivers on an individual basis?

Guidance: No, except upon request for resolution of a conflict of medical evaluations.

§391.49 Waiver of certain physical defects

Question 1: Since 49 CFR 391.49 does not mandate a Skill Performance Evaluation, does the term "performance standard" mean that the State must give a driving test or other Skill Performance Evaluation to the driver for every waiver issued or does this term mean that, depending upon the medical condition, the State may give some other type of performance test? For example, in the case of a vision waiver, would a vision examination suffice as a performance standard?

Guidance: Under the Tolerance Guidelines, Appendix C, Paragraph 3(j), each State that creates a waiver program for intrastate drivers is responsible for determining what constitutes "sound medical judgment," as well as determining the performance standard. In the example used above, a vision examination would suffice as a performance standard. It is the responsibility of each State establishing a waiver program to determine what constitutes an appropriate performance standard.

Schedules of Controlled Substances

§1308.11 Schedule I.

(a) Schedule I shall consist of the drugs and other substances, by whatever official name, common or usual name, chemical name, or brand name designated, listed in this section. Each drug or substance has been assigned the DEA Controlled Substances Code Number set forth opposite it.

IX. Reference

(b) **Opiates**. Unless specifically excepted or unless listed in another schedule, any of the following opiates, including their isomers, esters, ethers, salts, and salts of isomers, esters and ethers, whenever the existence of such isomers, esters, ethers and salts is possible within the specific chemical designation (for purposes of 3-methylthiofentanyl only, the term isomer includes the optical and geometric isomers):

336

REFERENCE

IX. Reference

338

REFERENCE

IX. Reference

(c) **Opium Derivatives**. Unless specifically excepted or unless listed in another schedule, any of the following opium derivatives, its salts, isomers, and salts of isomers whenever the existence of such salts, isomers, and salts of isomers is possible within the specific chemical designation:

(1)	Acetorphine	9319
(2)	Acetyldihydrocodeine	9051
(3)	Benzylmorphine	9052
(4)	Codeine methylbromide	9070
(5)	Codeine-N-Oxide	9053
(6)	Cyprenorphine	9054
(7)	Desomorphine	9055
(8)	Dihydromorphine	9145
(9)	Drotebanol	9335
(10)	Etorphine (except hydrochloride salt)	9056
(11)	Heroin	9200
(12)	Hydromorphinol	9301
(13)	Methyldesorphine	9302
(14)	Methyldihydromorphine	9304
(15)	Morphine methylbromide	9305
(16)	Morphine methylsulfonate	9306
(17)	Morphine-N-Oxide	9307
(18)	Myrophine	9308
(19)	Nicocodeine	9309
(20)	Nicomorphine	9312
(21)	Normorphine	9313
(22)	Pholcodine	9314
(23)	Thebacon	9315

(d) **Hallucinogenic substances.** Unless specifically excepted or unless listed in another schedule, any material, compound, mixture, or preparation, which contains any quantity of the following hallucinogenic substances, or which contains any of its salts, isomers, and salts of isomers whenever the existence of such salts, isomers, and salts of isomers is possible within the specific chemical designation (for purposes of this paragraph only, the term "isomer" includes the optical, position and geometric isomers):

(1) Alpha-ethyltryptamine
Some trade or other names: etryptamine; Monase; α-ethyl-1H-indole-3-ethanamine; 3-(2-aminobutyl) indole; α-ET; and AET.. 7249

(2) 4-bromo-2,5-dimethoxy-amphetamine
Some trade or other names: 4-bromo-2,5-dimethoxy-a-methylphenethylamine; 4-bromo-2,5-DMA.................... 7391

(3) 4-Bromo-2,5-dimethoxyphenethylamine
Some trade or other names: 2-(4-bromo-2,5-dimethoxyphenyl)-1-aminoethane; alpha-desmethyl DOB; 2C-B, Nexus. 7392

(4) 2,5-dimethoxyamphetamine
Some trade or other names: 2,5-dimethoxy-a-methylphenethylamine; 2.5-DMA.............................. 7396

(5) 2,5-dimethoxy-4-ethylamphetamine
Some trade or other names: DOET 7399

(6) 2,5-dimethoxy-4-(n)-propylthiophenethylamine (other name: 2C-T-7) 7348

(7) 4-methoxyamphetamine
Some trade or other names: 4-methoxy-a-methyl-phenethylamine; paramethoxyamphetamine, PMA 7411

(8) 5-methoxy-3,4-methylenedioxy-amphetamine 7401

(9) 4-methyl-2,5-dimethoxy-amphetamine
Some trade and other names: 4-methyl-2,5-dimethoxy-a-methylphenethylamine, "DOM"; and "STP" 7395

(10) 3,4-methylenedioxy amphetamine 7400

(11) 3,4-methylenedioxymethamphetamine (MDMA) 7405

(12) 3,4-methylenedioxy-N-ethylamphetamine (also known as N-ethyl-alpha-methyl-3,4 (methylenedioxy)phenethylamine, N-ethyl MDA, MDE, MDEA 7404

(13) N-hydroxy-3,4-methylenedioxyamphetamine (also known as N-hydroxy-alpha-methyl-3,4 (methylenedioxy) phenethylamine, and N-hydroxy MDA......................... 7402

(14) 3,4,5-trimethoxy amphetamine 7390

341

Meaning all parts of the plant presently classified botani-
cally as *Lophophora williams Lemaire,* whether growing or
not, the seeds thereof, any extract from any part of such
plant, and every compound, manufacture, salts, derivative,
mixture, or preparation of such plant, its seeds or extracts
(Interprets 21 USC 812(c), Schedule I(c) (12))

(i) Meaning tetrahydrocannabinols, except as in paragraph
(d)(31)(ii) of this section, naturally contained in a plant of
the genus Cannabis (cannabis plant), as well as synthetic
equivalents of the substances contained in the cannabis

plant, or in the resinous extractives of such plant, and/or synthetic substances, derivatives, and their isomers with similar chemical structure and pharmacological activity to those substances contained in the plant, such as the following:

> 1 cis or trans tetrahydrocannabinol, and their optical isomers
>
> 6 cis or trans tetrahydrocannabinol, and their optical isomers
>
> 3, 4 cis or trans tetrahydrocannabinol, and its optical isomers

(Since nomenclature of these substances is not internationally standardized, compounds of these structures, regardless of numerical designation of atomic positions covered.)

(ii) Tetrahydrocannabinols does not include any material, compound, mixture, or preparation that falls within the definition of hemp set forth in 7 U.S.C. 1639o.

IX. Reference

344

IX. Reference

(e) **Depressants**. Unless specifically excepted or unless listed in another schedule, any material, compound, mixture, or preparation which contains any quantity of the following substances having a depressant effect on the central nervous system, including its salts, isomers, and salts of isomers whenever the existence of such salts, isomers, and salts of isomers is possible within the specific chemical designation:

(f) **Stimulants.** Unless specifically excepted or unless listed in another schedule, any material, compound, mixture, or preparation which contains any quantity of the following substances having a stimulant effect on the central nervous system, including its salts, isomers, and salts of isomers:

(1) Aminorex (Some other names: aminoxaphen; 2-amino-5-phe-nyl-2-oxazoline; or 4,5-dehydro-5-phenly-2-oxazolamine).. 1585

(2) N-Benzylpiperazine (some other names: BZP, 1-benzylpiperazine) 7493

(3) Cathinone 1235
Some trade or other names: 2-amino-1-phenyl-1-propanone, alpha-aminopropiophenone, 2-aminopropiophenone, and norephedrone.

(4) (4) 4,4'-Dimethylaminorex (4,4'-DMAR; 4,5-dihydro-4-methyl-5-(4-methylphenyl)-2-oxazolamine; 4-methyl-5-(4-methylphenyl)-4,5-dihydro-1,3-oxazol-2-amine) 1595

(5) Fenthylline... 1503

(6) Methcathinone (Some other names: 2-(methylamino)-propiophenone; alpha-(methylamino)propiophenone; 2-(methylamino)-1-phenylpropan-1-one; alpha-*N*-methyl-aminopropiophenone; monomethylpropion; ephedrone; *N*-methylcathinone; methylcathinone; AL-464; AL-422; AL-463 and UR1432), its salts, optical isomers and salts of optical isomers.. 1237

(7) (±)*cis*-4-methylaminorex(±)*cis*-4,5-dihydro-4-methyl-5-phenyl-2-oxazolamine 1590

(8) N-ethylamphetamine.. 1475

(9) *N,N*-dimethylamphetamine (also known as *N,N*,alpha-trimethylbenzeneethanamine: *N,N*,alpha-trimethylphenethylamine)....................................... 1480

(g) **Cannabimimetic agents**. Unless specifically exempted or unless listed in another schedule, any material, compound, mixture, or preparation which contains any quantity of the following substances, or which contains their salts, isomers, and salts of isomers whenever the existence of such salts, isomers, and salts of isomers is possible within the specific chemical designation:

(1) 5-(1,1-dimethylheptyl)-2-[(1R,3S)-3-hydroxycyclohexyl]-phenol (CP-47,497) 7297

(2) 5-(1,1-dimethylheptyl)-2-[(1R,3S)-3-hydroxycyclohexyl]-phenol (cannabicyclohexanol or CP-47,497 C8-homolog)... 7298

(3) 1-pentyl-3-(1-naphthoyl)indole (JWH-018 and AM678)....... 7118

(4) 1-butyl-3-(1-naphthoyl)indole (JWH-073)...................... 7173

(5)   1-hexyl-3-(1-naphthoyl)indole (JWH-019) 7019

(6)   1-[2-(4-morpholinyl)ethyl]-3-(1-naphthoyl)indole (JWH-200) . 7200

(7)   1-pentyl-3-(2-methoxyphenylacetyl)indole (JWH-250) 6250

(8)   1-pentyl-3-[1-(4-methoxynaphthoyl)]indole (JWH-081) 7081

(9)   1-pentyl-3-(4-methyl-1-naphthoyl)indole (JWH-122) 7122

(10)   1-pentyl-3-(4-chloro-1-naphthoyl)indole (JWH-398)........... 7398

(11)   1-(5-fluoropentyl)-3-(1-naphthoyl)indole (AM2201) 7201

(12)   1-(5-fluoropentyl)-3-(2-iodobenzoyl)indole (AM694) 7694

(13)   1-pentyl-3-[(4-methoxy)-benzoyl]indole (SR-19 and RCS-
4) 7104

(14)   1-cyclohexylethyl-3-(2-methoxyphenylacetyl)indole 7008
(SR-18 and RCS-8) 7008

(15)   1-pentyl-3-(2-chlorophenylacetyl)indole (JWH-203)........... 7203

   (h) **Temporary listing of substances subject to emergency sched-
uling.** Any material, compound, mixture or preparation which contains
any quantity of the following substances:

(1) - [Reserved]
(29)

(30)   Fentanyl-related substances, their isomers, esters, ethers,
salts and salts of isomers, esters and ethers .... (9850)

   (i) Fentanyl-related substance means any substance not
   otherwise listed under another Administration Controlled
   Substance Code Number, and for which no exemption or
   approval is in effect under section 505 of the Federal
   Food, Drug, and Cosmetic Act [21 U.S.C. 355], that is
   structurally related to fentanyl by one or more of the following modifications:

      (A) Replacement of the phenyl portion of the phenethyl
      group by any monocycle, whether or not further substi-
      tuted in or on the monocycle;

      (B) Substitution in or on the phenethyl group with alkyl,
      alkenyl, alkoxyl, hydroxyl, halo, haloalkyl, amino or nitro
      groups;

      (C) Substitution in or on the piperidine ring with alkyl,
      alkenyl, alkoxyl, ester, ether, hydroxyl, halo, haloalkyl,
      amino or nitro groups;

      (D) Replacement of the aniline ring with any aromatic
      monocycle whether or not further substituted in or on
      the aromatic monocycle; and/or

(E) Replacement of the *N*-propionyl group by another acyl group.

(ii) This definition includes, but is not limited to, the following substances:

(A) [Reserved]

(B) [Reserved]

(31) [Reserved]
-
(41)

(42) *N*-Ethylhexedrone, its optical, positional, and geometric isomers, salts and salts of isomers (Other name: 2-(ethylamino)-1-phenylhexan-1-one) 7246

(43) *alpha*-Pyrrolidinohexanophenone, its optical, positional, and geometric isomers, salts and salts of isomers (Other names: α-PHP; *alpha*-pyrrolidinohexiophenone; 1-phenyl-2-(pyrrolidin-1-yl)hexan-1-one) 7544

(44) 4-Methyl-*alpha*-ethylaminopentiophenone, its optical, positional, and geometric isomers, salts and salts of isomers (Other names: 4-MEAP; 2-(ethylamino)-1-(4-methylphenyl)pentan-1-one) 7245

(45) 4'-Methyl-*alpha*-pyrrolidinohexiophenone, its optical, positional, and geometric isomers, salts and salts of isomers (Other names: MPHP; 4'-methyl-*alpha*-pyrrolidinohexanophenone; 1-(4-methylphenyl)-2-(pyrrolidin-1-yl)hexan-1-one).................................... 7446

(46) *alpha*-Pyrrolidinoheptaphenone, its optical, positional, and geometric isomers, salts and salts of isomers (Other names: PV8; 1-phenyl-2-(pyrrolidin-1-yl)heptan-1-one) 7548

(47) 4'-Chloro-*alpha*-pyrrolidinovalerophenone, its optical, positional, and geometric isomers, salts and salts of isomers (Other names: 4-chloro-α-PVP; 4'-chloro-*alpha*-pyrrolidinopentiophenone; 1-(4-chlorophenyl)-2-(pyrrolidin-1-yl)pentan-1-one) 7443

(48) [Removed and reserved]

(49) 1-(1-(1-(4-bromophenyl)ethyl)piperidin-4-yl)-1,3-dihydro-2H-benzo[d]imidazol-2-one, its isomers, esters, ethers, salts and salts of isomers, esters and ethers (Other names: brorphine; 1-[1-[1-(4-bromophenyl)ethyl]-4-piperidinyl]-1,3-dihydro-2H-benzimidazol-2- one) 9098

§1308.12 Schedule II

(a) Schedule II shall consist of the drugs and other substances, by whatever official name, common or usual name, chemical name, or brand name designated, listed in this section. Each drug or substance has been assigned the Controlled Substances Code Number set forth opposite it.

(b) **Substances, vegetable origin or chemical synthesis.** Unless specifically excepted or unless listed in another schedule, any of the following substances whether produced directly or indirectly by extraction from substances of vegetable origin, or independently by means of chemical synthesis, or by a combination of extraction and chemical synthesis:

(1) Opium and opiate, and any salt, compound, derivative, or preparation of opium or opiate excluding apomorphine, thebaine-derived butorphanol, dextrorphan, nalbuphine, naldemedine, nalmefene, naloxegol, naloxone, 6β-naltrexol, naltrexone, and samidorphan, and their respective salts, but including the following:

(i)	Codeine	9050
(ii)	Dihydroetorphine	9334
(iii)	Ethylmorphine	9190
(iv)	Etorphine hydrochloride	9059
(v)	Granulated opium	9640
(vi)	Hydrocodone	9193
(vii)	Hydromorphone	9150
(viii)	Metopon	9260
(ix)	Morphine	9300
(x)	Noroxymorphone	9668
(xi)	Opium extracts	9610
(xii)	Opium fluid	9620
(xiii)	Oripavine	9330
(xiv)	Oxycodone	9143
(xv)	Oxymorphone	9652
(xvi)	Powdered opium	9639
(xvii)	Raw opium	9600
(xviii)	Thebaine	9333
(xix)	Tincture of opium	9630

(2) Any salt, compound, derivative, or preparation thereof which is chemically equivalent or identical with any of the substances referred to in paragraph (b)(1) of this section, except that these substances shall not include the isoquinoline alkaloids of opium.

(3) Opium poppy and poppy straw.

(4) Coca leaves (9040) and any salt, compound, derivative or preparation of coca leaves (including cocaine (9041) and ecgonine (9180) and their salts, isomers, derivatives and salts of isomers and derivatives), and any salt, compound, derivative, or preparation thereof which is chemically equivalent or identical with any of these substances, except that the substances shall not include:

(i) Decocainized coca leaves or extraction of coca leaves, which extractions do not contain cocaine or ecgonine; or

(ii) [^{123}I]ioflupane.

(5) Concentrate of poppy straw (the crude extract of poppy straw in either liquid, solid or powder form which contains the phenanthrene alkaloids of the opium poppy), 9670.

(c) **Opiates.** Unless specifically excepted or unless in another schedule any of the following opiates, including its isomers, esters, ethers, salts and salts of isomers, esters and ethers whenever the existence of such isomers, esters, ethers, and salts is possible within the specific chemical designation, dextrorphan and levopropoxyphene excepted:

(1) Alfentanil 9737

IX. Reference

(d) **Stimulants.** Unless specifically excepted or unless listed in another schedule, any material, compound, mixture, or preparation which contains any quantity of the following substances having a stimulant effect on the central nervous system:

(1) Amphetamine, its salts, optical isomers, and salts of its optical isomers.. 1100

(2) Methamphetamine, its salts, isomers, and salts of its isomers.. 1105

(3) Phenmetrazine and its salts... 1631

(4) Methylphenidate 1724

(5) Lisdexamfetamine, its salts, isomers, and salts of its isomers .. 1205

(e) **Depressants.** Unless specifically excepted or unless listed in another schedule, any material, compound, mixture, or preparation which contains any quantity of the following substances having a depressant effect on the central nervous system, including its salts, isomers, and salts of isomers whenever the existence of such salts, isomers, and salts of isomers is possible within the specific chemical designation:

(1) Amobarbital.. 2125

(2) Glutethimide 2550

(3) Pentobarbital 2270

(4) Phencyclidine.. 7471

(5) Secobarbital 2315

(f) **Hallucinogenic substances.**

(1) Nabilone
[Another name of nabilone (-) *trans* 3-(1-1-dimethylheptyl) 6, 6a, 7, 8, 10, 10a hexahydro-1-hydroxy 6, 6-dimethyl 9H dibenzo(b d)pyran-9-one].. 7379

(2) Dronabinol [(-)-delta-9-*trans* tetrahydrocannabinol] in an oral solution in a drug product approved for marketing by the U.S. Food and Drug Administration .... (7365)

(g) **Immediate precursors.** Unless specifically excepted or unless listed in another schedule, any material, compound, mixture, or preparation which contains any quantity of the following substances:
(1) Immediate precursor to amphetamine and methamphetamine:

(i) Phenylacetone
Some trade or other names: phenyl-2-propanone; P2P; benzyl methyl ketone; methyl benzyl ketone;............................. 8501

(2) Immediate precursors to phenyclidine (PCP):

(i) 1-phenylcyclohexylamine 7460

(ii) 1-piperidinocyclohexanecarbonitrile (PCC)......................... 8603

(3) Immediate precursor to fentanyl:

(i) 4-anilino-N-phenethylpiperidine (ANPP) 8333

(ii) N-phenyl-N-(piperidin-4-yl)propionamide (norfentanyl)............ 8366

§1308.13 Schedule III.

(a) Schedule III shall consist of the drugs and other substances, by whatever official name, common or usual name, chemical name, or brand name designated, listed in this section. Each drug or substance has been assigned the DEA Controlled substances Code Number set forth opposite it.

(b) **Stimulants.** Unless specifically excepted or unless listed in another schedule, any material, compound, mixture, or preparation which contains any quantity of the following substances having a stimulant effect on the central nervous system, including its salts, isomers (whether optical, positional, or geometric), and salts of such isomers whenever the existence of such salts, isomers, and salts of isomers is possible within the specific chemical designation:

(1) Those compounds, mixtures, or preparations in dosage unit form containing any stimulant substances listed in schedule II which compounds, mixtures, or preparations were listed on August 25, 1971, as excepted compounds under §1308.32, and any other drug of the quantitive composition shown in that list for those drugs or which is the same except that it contains a lesser quantity of controlled substances 1405

(2) Benzphetamine 1228

(3) Chlorphentermine... 1645

(4) Clortermine 1647

(5) Phendimetrazine... 1615

(c) **Depressants.** Unless specifically excepted or unless listed in another schedule, any material, compound, mixture, or preparation which contains any quantity of the following substances having a depressant effect on the central nervous system:

(1) Any compound, mixture or preparation containing:

(i) Amobarbital.. 2126

(ii) Secobarbital 2316

(iii) Pentobarbital 2271

or any salt thereof and one or more other active medicinal ingredients which are not listed in any schedule.

(2) Any suppository dosage form containing:

(i) Amobarbital.. 2126

(ii) Secobarbital 2316

(iii) Pentobarbital .... 2271 or any salt of any of these drugs and approved by the Food and Drug Administration for marketing only as a suppository.

(3)   Any substance which contains any quantity of a derivative of barbituric acid or any salt thereof............................ 2100

(4)   Chlorhexadol... 2510

(5)   Embutramide 2020

(6)   Any drug product containing gamma hydroxybutyric acid, including its salts, isomers, and salts of isomers, for which an application is approved under section 505 of the Federal Food, Drug, and Cosmetic Act............................ 2012

(7)   Ketamine, its salts, isomers, and salts of isomers [Some other names for ketamine: (±)-2-(2-chlorophenyl)-2-(methylamino)-cyclohexanone]. 7285

(8)   Lysergic acid... 7300

(9)   Lysergic acid amide... 7310

(10) Methyprylon... 2575

(11) Perampanel, and its salts, isomers, and salts of isomers ... 2261

(12) Sulfondiethylmethane.. 2600

(13) Sulfonethylmethane... 2605

(14) Sulfonmethane 2610

(15) Tiletamine and zolazepam or any salt thereof 7295

Some trade or other names for a tiletaminezolazepan combination product: Telazol

Some trade or other names for tiletamine: 2-(ethylamino)-2-(2-thienyl)-cyclohexanone

Some trade or other names for zolazepam: 4-(2-fluorophenyl)-6,8-dihydro-1,3,8-trimethylpyrazolo-[3,4-e] [1,4]-diazepin-7(1H)-one, flupyrazapon

(d) Nalorphine 9400.

(e) **Narcotic drugs.** Unless specifically excepted or unless listed in another schedule:

(1)   Any material, compound, mixture, or preparation containing any of the following narcotic drugs, or their salts calculated as the free anhydrous base or alkaloid, in limited quantities as set forth below:

(i)   Not more than 1.8 grams of codeine per 100 milliliters or not more than 90 milligrams per dosage unit, with an equal or greater quantity of an isoquinoline alkaloid of opium 9803

(f) **Anabolic steroids.** Unless specifically excepted or unless listed in another schedule, any material, compound, mixture, or preparation, containing any quantity of the following substances, including its salts, esters and ethers:

    (g) **Hallucinogenic substances.**

§1308.14 Schedule IV.

(a) Schedule IV shall consist of the drugs and other substances, by whatever official name, common or usual name, chemical name, or brand name designated, listed in this section. Each drug or substance has been assigned the DEA Controlled Substances Code Number set forth opposite it.

(b) **Narcotic drugs.** Unless specifically excepted or unless listed in another schedule, any material, compound, mixture, or preparation containing any of the following narcotic drugs, or their salts calculated as the free anhydrous base or alkaloid, in limited quantities as set forth below:

(1) Not more than 1 milligram of difenoxin and not less than 25 micrograms of atropine sulfate per dosage unit 9167
(2) Dextropopoxyphene (alpha-(+)-4-dimethylamino-1,2-diphenyl-3-methyl-2-propionoxybutane) 9278
(3) 2-[(dimethylamino)methyl]-1-(3-methoxyphenyl)cyclohexanol, its salts, optical and geometric isomers and salts of these isomers (including tramadol).. 9752

(c) **Depressants.** Unless specifically excepted or unless listed in another schedule, any material, compound, mixture, or preparation which contains any quantity of the following substances, including its salts, isomers, and salts of isomers whenever the existence of such salts, isomers, and salts of isomers is possible within the specific chemical designation:

(1)	Alfaxalone	2731
(2)	Alprazolam	2882
(3)	Barbital	2145
(4)	Brexanolone	2400
(5)	Bromazepam	2748
(6)	Camazepam	2749
(7)	Carisoprodol	8192
(8)	Chloral betaine	2460
(9)	Chloral hydrate	2465
(10)	Chlordiazepoxide	2744
(11)	Clobazam	2751
(12)	Clonazepam	2737
(13)	Clorazepate	2768
(14)	Clotiazepam	2752
(15)	Cloxazolam	2753
(16)	Daridorexant	2410
(17)	Delorazepam	2754
(18)	Diazepam	2765
(19)	Dichloralphenazone	2467
(20)	Estazolam	2756
(21)	Ethchlorvynol	2540
(22)	Ethinamate	2545

(d) **Fenfluramine.** Any material, compound, mixture, or preparation which contains any quantity of the following substances, including its salts, isomers (whether optical, position, or geometric), and salts of such isomers, whenever the existence of such salts, isomers, and salts of isomers is possible:

(1) Fenfluramine 1670

(e) **Lorcaserin.** Any material, compound, mixture, or preparation which contains any quantity of the following substances, including its salts, isomers, and salts of such isomers, whenever the existence of such salts, isomers, and salts of isomers is possible:

(1) Lorcaserin... 1625

(f) **Stimulants.** Unless specifically excepted or unless listed in another schedule, any material, compound, mixture, or preparation which contains any quantity of the following substances having a stimulant effect on the central nervous system, including its salts, isomers and salts of isomers:

(1)	Cathine ((+)-norpseudophedrine)	1230
(2)	Diethylpropion	1610
(3)	Fencamfamin	1760
(4)	Fenproporex	1575
(5)	Mazindol	1605
(6)	Mefenorex	1580
(7)	Modafinil	1680
(8)	Pemoline (including organometallic complexes and chelates thereof)	1530
(9)	Phentermine	1640
(10)	Pipradrol	1750
(11)	Serdexmethylphenidate	1729
(12)	Sibutramine	1675
(13)	Solriamfetol (2-amino-3-phenylpropyl car-bamate; benzenepropanol, betaamino-, carbamate (ester))	1650
(14)	SPA ((-)-1-dimethylamino-1,2-diphenylethane)	1635

(g) **Other substances.** Unless specifically excepted or unless listed in another schedule, any material, compound, mixture or preparation which contains any quantity of the following substances, including its salts:

(1) Pentazocine 9709
(2) Butorphanol... 9720

§1308.15 Schedule V.

(a) Schedule V shall consist of the drugs and other substances, by whatever official name, common or usual name, chemical name or brand name designated, listed in this section.

(b) **Narcotic drugs.** Unless specifically excepted or unless listed in another schedule, any material, compound, mixture, or preparation containing any of the following narcotic drugs and their salts, as set forth below:

(1) [Reserved]

(c) **Narcotic drugs containing nonnarcotic active medicinal ingredients.** Any compound, mixture, or preparation containing any of the following narcotic drugs, or their salts calculated as the free anhydrous base or alkaloid, in limited quantities as set forth below, which shall include one or more non-narcotic active medicinal ingredients in sufficient proportion to confer upon the compound, mixture, or preparation valuable medicinal qualities other than those possessed by narcotic drugs alone:

(1) Not more than 200 milligrams of codeine per 100 milliliters or per 100 grams.

(2) Not more than 100 milligrams of dihydrocodeine per 100 milliliters or per 100 grams.

(3) Not more than 100 milligrams of ethylmorphine per 100 milliliters or per 100 grams.

(4) Not more than 2.5 milligrams of diphenoxylate and not less than 25 micrograms of atropine sulfate per dosage unit.

(5) Not more than 100 milligrams of opium per 100 milliliters or per 100 grams.

(6) Not more than 0.5 milligram of difenoxin and not less than 25 micrograms of atropine sulfate per dosage unit.

(d) **Stimulants.** Unless specifically exempted or excluded or unless listed in another schedule, any material, compound, mixture, or preparation which contains any quantity of the following substances having a stimulant effect on the central nervous system, including its salts, isomers and salts of isomers:

(1) Pyrovalerone 1485

(2) [Reserved]

(e) **Depressants.** Unless specifically exempted or excluded or unless listed in another schedule, any material, compound, mixture, or preparation which contains any quantity of the following substances having a depressant effect on the central nervous system, including its salts:

(1) Brivaracetam ((2S)-2-[(4R)-2-oxo-4-propylpyrrolidin-1-yl] butanamide) (also referred to as BRV; UCB-34714; Briviact) (including its salts)... 2710

REFERENCE

FMCSA Bulletin: Obstructive Sleep Apnea

> **NOTE:** The FMCSA issued the following bulletin to medical examiners and training organizations in January 2015.

The purpose of this bulletin is to remind healthcare professionals on FMCSA's National Registry of Certified Medical Examiners (the National Registry) of the current physical qualifications standard and advisory criteria concerning the respiratory system, specifically how the requirements apply to drivers that may have obstructive sleep apnea (OSA).

Current Physical Qualifications Standard for Respiratory Conditions

FMCSA's physical qualifications standards prohibit individuals from receiving a medical examiner's certificate to operate commercial motor vehicles in interstate commerce if they have an "established medical history or clinical diagnosis of a respiratory dysfunction likely to interfere with his or her ability to control and drive a commercial motor vehicle safely." (49 CFR 391.41(b)(5)). OSA is considered a respiratory dysfunction when there is a determination that it is likely to interfere with the driver's ability to operate safely because of the severity of the case.

OSA is a respiratory disorder characterized by a reduction or cessation of breathing during sleep coupled with symptoms such as excessive daytime sleepiness. Given this, OSA may culminate in unpredictable and sudden incapacitation (e.g., falling asleep at the wheel), thus contributing to the potential for crashes, injuries, and fatalities.

During sleep, OSA blocks the airway and prevents the individual from breathing up to dozens of times per hour, awakening the sleeper. This means that the time in bed does not equal time slept – in fact, eight hours of sleep with OSA can be less refreshing than four hours of ordinary, uninterrupted sleep, posing serious cognitive and neuropsychological risks. Moreover, someone without enough restorative sleep is often unaware of impairments to a range of cognitive abilities such as vigilance, reaction time, attention span, memory, learning, problem-solving, decision making, and multitasking. OSA can also lead to mood swings and difficulty controlling inappropriate feelings. In driving simulations, OSA patients were more likely to unintentionally swerve and strike objects – a serious and dangerous outcome for the transportation industry.

OSA raises health and safety concerns beyond those of other sleep disorders. Near-term increases in fatigue and cognitive dysfunction can result. Also, there are long-term adverse health effects such as dramatically increased risk for hypertension, heart disease, stroke, diabetes, and obesity.

FMCSA's Advisory Criteria from 2000

In 2000, FMCSA issued advisory criteria providing interpretive guidance to medical examiners concerning its physical qualifications standards. These advisory criteria are recommendations from FMCSA to assist medical examiners in applying the minimum physical qualification standards. The advisory criteria have been published with the Federal Motor Carrier Safety Regulations as part of the medical examination report form in 49 CFR 391.43 (Physical Qualification of Drivers; Medical Examination; Certificate, 65 FR 59363 (October 5, 2000)).

The advisory criterion for §391.41(b)(5), which has been unchanged since 2000, provides the following guidance for medical examiners in making the determination whether a driver satisfies the respiratory standard:

Since a driver must be alert at all times, any change in his or her mental state is in direct conflict with highway safety. Even the slightest impairment in respiratory function under emergency conditions (when greater oxygen supply is necessary for performance) may be detrimental to safe driving.

There are many conditions that interfere with oxygen exchange and may result in incapacitation, including emphysema, chronic asthma, carcinoma, tuberculosis, chronic bronchitis and sleep apnea. If the medical examiner detects a respiratory dysfunction, that in any way is likely to interfere with the driver's ability to safely control and drive a commercial motor vehicle, the driver must be referred to a specialist for further evaluation and therapy. Anticoagulation therapy for deep vein thrombosis and/or pulmonary thromboembolism is not unqualifying once optimum dose is achieved, provided lower extremity venous examinations remain normal and the treating physician gives a favorable recommendation.

Based on the above advisory criterion, it is clear that FMCSA has considered OSA a respiratory dysfunction that interferes with oxygen exchange. And the Agency recommends that, if a medical examiner believes the driver's respiratory condition is in any way likely to interfere with the driver's ability to safely control and drive a commercial motor vehicle, the driver should be referred to a specialist for further evaluation and therapy. This advisory criterion is helpful to medical examiners when the examiner has sufficient experience or information to recognize certain risk factors for OSA, or when a driver tells the examiner that he or she has been diagnosed with OSA. Under these circumstances, the medical examiner should consider referring the driver to a specialist for evaluation before issuing a medical examiner's certificate, or request additional information from the driver and his or her treating healthcare professional about the management of the driver's OSA, respectively.

Role of Medical Examiners' Clinical Judgment in the Medical Certification Process

FMCSA's physical qualifications standards and advisory criteria do not provide OSA screening, diagnosis or treatment guidelines for medical examiners to use in determining whether an individual should be issued a medical certificate. Medical examiners may exercise their medical judgment and expertise in determining whether a driver exhibits risk factors for having OSA and in determining whether additional information is needed before making a decision whether to issue the driver a medical certificate and the duration of that medical certification.

FMCSA urges medical examiners to explain clearly to drivers the basis for their decision concerning the issuance of a medical certification for a period of less than two years or the denial of a medical certification. The Agency encourages medical examiners to consider the following in making the medical certification decision:

- The primary safety goal regarding OSA is to identify drivers with moderate-to-severe OSA to ensure these drivers are managing their condition to reduce to the greatest extent practical the risk of drowsy driving. Moderate-to-severe OSA is defined by an apnea-hypopnea index (AHI)[1] of greater than or equal to 15.

- The Agency does not require that these drivers be considered unfit to continue their driving careers; only that the medical examiner make a determination whether they need to be evaluated and, if warranted, demonstrate they are managing their OSA to reduce the risk of drowsy driving.

- ***Screening:*** With regard to identifying drivers with undiagnosed OSA, FMCSA's regulations and advisory criteria do not include screening guidelines. Medical examiners should consider common OSA symptoms such as loud snoring, witnessed apneas, or sleepiness during the major wake periods, as well as risk factors, and consider multiple risk factors such as body mass index (BMI), neck size, involvement in a single-vehicle crash, etc.

- ***Diagnosis:*** Methods of diagnosis include in-laboratory polysomnography, at-home polysomnography, or other limited channel ambulatory testing devices which ensure chain of custody.

- ***Treatment:*** OSA is a treatable condition, and drivers with moderate-to-severe OSA can manage the condition effectively to reduce the risk of drowsy driving. Treatment options range from weight loss to dental appliances to Continuous Positive Airway Pressure (CPAP) therapy, and combinations of these treatments. The Agency's regulations and advisory criteria do not include recommendations for treatments for OSA and FMCSA believes the issue of treatment is best left to the treating healthcare professional and the driver.

Conclusion

FMCSA relies on medical examiners to make driver qualification decisions based on their clinical observations, findings and standards of practice. The current regulations and advisory criteria do not include guidelines concerning OSA screening, diagnosis and treatment. Medical examiners should rely upon their medical training and expertise in determining whether a driver exhibits symptoms and/or multiple risk factors

[1] AHI = (apneas + hypopneas)/hours of sleep. Apnea is a term for the involuntary suspension of breathing during sleep. During an apnea there is no movement of the respiratory muscles and the volume of air in the lungs initially remains unchanged. Hypopnea is a term for a disorder which involves episodes of overly shallow breathing or an abnormally low respiratory rate. This differs from apnea in that there remains some flow of air. Hypopnea events may happen while asleep or while awake.

for OSA, and they should explain to the driver the basis
for their decision if the examiner decides to issue a
medical certificate for a period of less than two years to
allow for further evaluation, or to deny a driver the
medical certificate.

FAQs

General

What medical conditions disqualify a commercial bus or truck driver?

The truck driver must be medically qualified to not only
drive the vehicle safely, but also to do pre- and post-trip
safety inspections, secure the load, and make sure it
has not shifted. Bus drivers have different demands.

By regulation, specific medically disqualifying conditions found under §391.41 are hearing loss, vision loss
(except as allowed under §391.44), epilepsy, and insulin
use (except as allowed under §391.46). For other conditions, the medical examiner can use his/her judgment to
determine the conditions under which the driver may
be qualified, taking into consideration all the clinical
evidence as well as the FMCSA's medical guidelines,
recommendations, and regulations.

Drivers who require a diabetes or vision exemption to
safely drive a CMV in addition to those pre-printed on
the certification form are disqualified until they receive
such an exemption.

Why is the DOT physical examination important?

The FMCSA physical examination is required to help
ensure that a person is medically qualified to safely operate a CMV. In the interest of public safety, CMV drivers are held to higher physical, mental, and emotional
standards than passenger car drivers.

Is the employer legally responsible for paying for the DOT medical examination?

The FMCSRs do not address this issue.

Are the DOT medical examinations covered by HIPAA?

Regulatory requirements take precedence over the *Health Insurance Portability and Accountability Act* (HIPAA) of 1996. There are potential subtle interpretations that can cause significant problems for the medical examiner. What information must or can be turned over to the carrier is a legal issue, and if in doubt, the examiner should obtain a legal opinion. Federal Motor Carrier Safety Regulation §391.43 does not address or prohibit the sharing of medical information by medical examiners. See http://www.hhs.gov/ocr/hipaa

Does the FMCSA set any guidelines for medical examiner fees associated with conducting medical examinations?

No. There is no fee schedule.

Does my driving record affect my eligibility for a medical certificate?

No.

Are CMV drivers required to be CPR certified?

No. There is no regulation that requires CMV drivers to be CPR certified.

Does a driver need a new physical when he/she returns to work after a medical leave?

Any driver who has received physical or mental injury or disease which has impaired his/her ability to perform normal duties must have a physical examination and obtain a new medical examiner's certificate. However, if a driver returns from a medical leave, a new physical is not necessarily required unless the employer questions the driver's abilities to perform his/her job duties. If the driver has a current, valid medical certificate, a motor carrier can continue to accept this card if the driver's abilities are not in question.

367

Are motor carriers legally obligated to provide air conditioning in commercial motor vehicles?

The FMCSRs do not address this issue.

If an examiner disqualifies a driver due to a medical concern, can the driver go to another doctor for a new physical, in hopes of being certified?

The FMCSA regulations do not currently prohibit this practice. However, through its National Registry, the FMCSA receives reports about the drivers who have been certified, and by whom, and the agency may investigate specific drivers or examiners. Conflicts that arise between two examiners should be resolved under the procedures in §391.47 (see Chapter 7).

Can a driver's medical examiner be located in a different state than the one in which the driver is licensed, or in which the driver lives?

Yes. There are no restrictions placed on the location of the examiner.

Does a driver who is required to wear corrective lenses need to have a spare set of lenses in the vehicle?

No. Though recommended, there is no such requirement under FMCSA rules. The driver must be wearing corrective lenses while driving if such a restriction is on the driver's license and/or medical card.

Does a driver who is required to wear a hearing aid need a spare power source in the vehicle?

No. Though recommended, there is no such requirement under FMCSA rules (although there used to be).

Do employers have access to a driver's medical evaluation?

Although the FMCSRs do not require the medical examiner to give a copy of the Medical Examination Report to the employer, the FMCSA does not prohibit employers from obtaining copies of the medical examination form (long form). Medical examiners should have a release form signed by the driver if the employer wishes to obtain a copy of the form.

Employers must comply with applicable state and federal laws regarding the privacy and maintenance of employee medical information. For information about the provisions of the Standards for Privacy of Individually Identifiable Health Information (the Privacy Rule) that was mandated by the *Health Insurance Portability & Accountability Act of 1996* (HIPAA) (Public Law 104-191), contact the U.S. Department of Health & Human Services at the HIPAA website of the Office of Civil Rights. Their toll-free information line is: (866) 627-7748.

What information should the medical examiner have available to decide if a driver is medically qualified?

Medical examiners who perform FMCSA medical examinations should understand:

1. Specific physical and mental demands associated with operating a CMV,

2. Physical qualification standards specified by 49 CFR §391.41(b)(1-13),

3. FMCSA advisory criteria and other criteria prepared by the FMCSA, and

4. FMCSA medical guidelines to assess the CMV driver's medical condition.

How do medical examiners differ from Medical Review Officers?

A Medical Review Officer (MRO) is a licensed physician responsible for receiving and reviewing laboratory results generated by an employer's drug testing program and evaluating medical explanations for test results. More information on MROs is available online at http://www.dot.gov/ost/dapc/mro.html. Medical Examiner means a person who is licensed, certified, or registered, in accordance with applicable state laws and regulations to perform physical examinations.

As a medical examiner, can I disclose the results of my medical evaluation to a CMV driver's employer?

Section 391.43 does not address or prohibit the sharing of medical information. Refer to the HIPAA regulations for guidance: http://www.hhs.gov/ocr/hipaa

What happens if a driver is not truthful about his/her health history on the medical examination form?

The FMCSA medical certification process is designed to ensure drivers are physically qualified to operate commercial vehicles safely. Each driver is required to complete the Health History section on the first page of the examination report and certify that the responses are complete and true. The driver must also certify that he/she understands that inaccurate, false or misleading information may invalidate the examination and medical examiner's certificate.

FMCSA relies on the medical examiner's clinical judgment to decide whether additional information should be obtained from the driver's treating physician. Deliberate omission or falsification of information may invalidate the examination and any certificate issued based on it. A civil penalty may also be levied against the driver under 49 U.S.C. 521(b)(2)(b), either for making a false statement of – or concealing – a disqualifying condition.

Alcohol

If the driver admits to regular alcohol use, and based on responses on the driver history, further questioning, or additional tools such as CAGE, AUDIT, or TWEAK assessments, may the examiner require further evaluation prior to signing the medical certificate?

Yes. As with most medical conditions, the final determination as to whether the driver meets the FMCSA medical standards for alcoholism is to be made by the medical examiner. The examiner should use whatever tools or additional assessments they feel are necessary. Under §391.43, support is provided to the examiner if they believe that "Other test(s) may be indicated based upon the medical history or findings of the physical examination."

Further supporting the need for additional evaluation is the medical advisory criteria for §391.41(b)(13) which notes that "if an individual shows signs of having an alcohol-use problem, he or she should be referred to a specialist. After counseling and/or treatment, he or she may be considered for certification."

The medical advisory criteria in Appendix A to Part 391 are provided by the FMCSA to help the examiner determine if a person is physically qualified to operate a CMV. The examiner may or may not choose to use these guidelines. These guidelines are based on expert review and considered practice standards. The examiner should document the reason(s) for not following the guidelines.

Medical Certificate

My medical certificate is still valid. Am I prohibited from operating a CMV if I have a medical condition that developed after my last medical certificate was issued?

FMCSA regulations prohibit a driver from beginning or continuing to drive if their ability and/or alertness is

REFERENCE

impaired by: fatigue, illness, or any cause that makes it unsafe to begin (or continue) to drive a commercial vehicle.

Even if a driver currently has a valid medical certificate, the driver is prohibited from driving a CMV with any medical condition that would be disqualifying or may interfere with the safe operation of a CMV. Once a disqualifying medical condition is resolved, and before resuming operation of CMVs, a driver is responsible for obtaining re-certification from a Medical Examiner (see §391.45).

What is the protocol if the medical certificate gets damaged, lost, or unreadable?

A copy of the Medical Examiner's Certificate should be kept on file in the medical examiner's office. The driver may request a replacement copy of the certificate from the medical examiner or get a copy of the certificate from the motor carrier.

How can I get a copy of my medical evaluation file?

You can contact the medical examiner that conducted your evaluation for a copy of your medical certification examination

I lost my medical card. What if the certifying doctor is no longer available?

If the original medical examiner is not available, the physician or medical examiner in the office may sign the replacement certificate. The advisory criteria states that the original may be copied and given to the driver. Some physicians may require the driver to undergo a new physical examination.

If a new driver has a current medical card from a previous employer, can the new employer accept it?

Yes. However, the carrier is not obligated to accept the certificate and may send the driver for a new physical.

Do drivers need to carry a copy of the long physical exam form in the vehicle?

No, drivers are not required to have a copy of the long DOT physical examination form. Drivers are only responsible for carrying a legible copy of the medical examiner's certificate and medical variance documentation, when required.

Is a release form required to be completed in order for the employer to legally keep the medical certification card on file?

No. The Medical Examiner is required to provide a copy of the Medical Examiner's Certificate (§391.43(g)) to any prospective or currently employing motor carrier who requests it. A release form is not required. In many cases, the motor carrier is required to keep a copy of the certificate in the driver qualification file (§391.51(b)).

Is the certification limited to current employment or job duties?

When a medical examiner grants medical certification, he/she certifies the driver to perform any job duty required of a commercial driver, not just the driver's current job duties.

Does a driver need a valid medical card to perform a road test?

If the vehicle is a "commercial motor vehicle" as defined in §390.5, then a valid medical card (and driver's license) is required.

If a driver moves, does the address on the medical card need to be updated?

No, there are no requirements for updating the address prior to the next exam.

If an exam is put into "Determination Pending" status, can the driver continue to drive?

Yes, but only if the driver still holds a valid medical card. A "pending" status means the certification decision could not be completed. The driver must rely on his/her *existing* medical card (if any) to continue to drive. If that card expires before the new certification decision can be completed, then the driver is no longer qualified.

If a driver receives a short-term medical card (30 days, 60 days, 6 months, etc.), does the driver need an entirely new medical exam once the short-term card expires?

Yes, once an examiner completes an exam, makes a certification decision (for any length of time), and issues a certificate to the driver, the examiner may not issue another certificate at a later date — or extend the original expiration date — without completing an entirely new exam.

If a driver's medical card does not expire for another 30 days but he/she goes for a new exam and is not issued a new certificate (i.e., is disqualified), does the old medical card remain valid until its expiration?

The results of the new exam supersede the existing certification, making the old card invalid.

Who signs the medical certificate?

The medical examiner who performs the medical examination must sign the certificate.

Who is required to have a copy of the medical certificate?

Section 391.43(g) requires the medical examiner to give a copy of the medical certificate to the driver and (upon request) the motor carrier, if the driver passes the medical examination. For drivers holding a commercial driver's license and operating in interstate commerce, a copy must also be provided to the state licensing agency.

May I request reconsideration if I am found not qualified for a medical certificate?

The decision to qualify a driver to operate a CMV in interstate commerce is the sole responsibility of the medical examiner. The driver may discuss the basis for the disqualification with the medical examiner and explore options for reconsideration.

For how long is a medical certificate valid?

The certificate is valid for a maximum of 2 years. Drivers with specific medical conditions, however, require more frequent certification. The length of certification is generally left to the examiner's discretion, but there are guidelines for specific conditions including:

- Hypertension (high blood pressure) stable on treatment: 1 year

- Heart disease: 1 year

- Qualified under §391.46 or §391.64: 1 year

- Vision exemption program: 1 year

- Driving in exempt intra-city zone: 1 year

Are holders of Class 3 pilot licenses required to have another physical for commercial driving?

Drivers of CMVs who operate in interstate commerce must be medically qualified in accordance with 49 CFR §391.41

Can carriers set their own medical standards for CMV drivers who operate in interstate commerce?

Section 390.3(d) gives employers the right to adopt stricter medical standards. Motor carriers cannot set less restrictive standards. In addition, the employer can require the driver to perform ancillary duties as a condition of employment.

What are the differences between the medical standards and the medical advisory criteria and the medical guidelines?

The medical examiner must follow the standards found in §391.41. In the case of vision, hearing, and epilepsy, the FMCSR standards are absolute and allow no discretion by the medical examiner, although drivers may be able to apply for an exemption.

FMCSA also provides medical advisory criteria and medical guidelines to assist the medical examiner determine if a person is physically qualified to operate a commercial bus or truck. The examiner may or may not choose to use these guidelines. These guidelines are based on expert review and considered practice standards. The examiner should document the reason(s) for not following the guidelines.

How long does it take to get my medical certificate once my medical examination is complete?

The FMCSRs do not specify that the medical examiner must give a copy of the Medical Examiner's Certificate to the driver immediately following the examination. The medical examiner may require additional medical tests or reports from the treating physician. An exam may remain in "pending" status for up to 45 days.

Can I still get a medical certificate if I have a medical condition that is being treated by a physician?

The decision is made by the medical examiner. The examiner may request information about the driver's condition from their treating doctor. In general, certification is permitted if the driver does not have a condition, use medication, or receive treatment that impairs safe driving.

As a medical examiner, can I disclose the results of my medical evaluation to a CMV driver's employer?

FMCSA regulations do not address or prohibit the sharing of medical information. Refer to the HIPAA regulations for guidance: http://www.hhs.gov/ocr/hipaa

Is the driver required to provide a copy to the employer?

Yes, the motor carrier (employer) is required to keep a copy of the medical card (certificate) on file. The copy may also be obtained directly from the medical examiner. In the case of CDL/CLP drivers, the card must only be retained for 15 days, although a 3-year retention period is recommended.

Can I report a driver operating without a medical certificate? What protection can I expect as a whistleblower and to whom would I report it?

Yes. Reports can be made by telephone to (888) DOT-SAFT (368-7238). For details on whistleblower protections, see www.whistleblowers.gov.

Am I required to have a medical certificate if I only operate a CMV in my home state (intrastate commerce)?

Intrastate drivers are subject to the physical qualification regulations of their states. All 50 states have adapted their regulations based on some of the federal requirements. Many states grant waivers for certain medical conditions. NOTE: Drivers for private package delivery services usually do not leave the state but are usually subject to interstate (federal) regulations.

Are government employees exempt from routine/ yearly physical examinations?

Transportation performed by the federal government, a state, or any political subdivision of a state, or an agency established under a compact between states that has been approved by the Congress of the United States are exempt from the FMCSRs, if the political entity chooses.

Is getting a medical certificate mandatory for all CMV drivers in the United States?

In general, all CMV drivers driving in interstate commerce within the United States must obtain medical certification from a medical examiner. CMV drivers from Canada and Mexico can be medically qualified in their countries.

I operate a CMV in the United States but reside outside of the United States. Can I use my foreign medical certificate?

Yes, if you are a resident of Mexico or Canada. Drivers certified in Canada are certified to drive in the United States, providing they meet U.S. requirements. For Mexican drivers, the medical examination is part of the *Licencia Federal*. It is not necessary for Mexican drivers to carry a separate medical certifying document.

A CMV operator from Canada or Mexico who has been issued a valid commercial driver's license by a Canadian Province or the Mexican *Licencia Federal* is no longer required to have a medical certificate. The driver's medical exam is part of the driver's license process and is proof of medical fitness to drive in the United States. However, Canadian and Mexican drivers who are insulin-using diabetics, who have epilepsy, or who are hearing-and-vision impaired are not qualified to drive CMVs in the United States. Furthermore, Canadian drivers who do not meet the medical fitness provisions of the Canadian National Safety Code for Motor Carriers but who have been issued a waiver by one of the Canadian Provinces or Territories are not qualified to drive CMVs in the United States. Similarly, Mexican drivers who do not meet the medical fitness provision of the *Licencia Federal de Conductor* but who have been issued a waiver by the *Licencia Federal de Conductor* are not qualified to drive CMVs in the United States.

Can a Canadian driver apply for a Skill Performance Evaluation (SPE) certificate to drive in the United States?

The reciprocity agreement between the United States and Canada does not permit drivers who do not meet the medical fitness requirements of Canada to drive in the United States. Both countries agree that Canadian drivers who do not meet the medical provisions in the National Safety Code of Canada but have a waiver by one of the Canadian Provinces or territories would not be qualified to operate a CMV in the United States. The National Safety Code states that a driver must wear a prosthesis and demonstrate his/her ability in an on-road test. Some of the Canadian provinces have not adopted the National Safety Code. If a driver has no prosthesis when entering the United States., the driver is not qualified to operate here.

It is not necessary for a Canadian driver to apply for a Skill Performance Evaluation certificate to drive in the United States. A valid commercial driver's license issued by a Canadian Province or Territory is proof of medical fitness to drive. If a Canadian driver is required to wear prosthesis, the driver must wear the prosthesis while operating a commercial vehicle in the U.S. If a driver has no prosthesis when entering the U.S., the driver is not qualified to operate here.

Medications

Does the FMCSA have a list of prohibited drugs?

Except in the case of a few drugs like methadone, marijuana, insulin, and Schedule I controlled substances, the FMCSA does not have a list of specific medications that drivers cannot take and remain qualified. In most cases, medical examiners have discretion to prescribe medications for therapeutic purposes. The medical examiner must decide if the driver can be medically certified to drive while taking the medication.

Can CMV drivers be qualified while being prescribed Provigil (Modafinil)?

Provigil (Modafinil) is a medication used to treat excessive sleepiness caused by certain sleep disorders. These sleep disorders are narcolepsy, obstructive sleep apnea/ hypopnea syndrome, and shift-work sleep disorders. Provigil has several concerning side effects such as chest pain, dizziness, difficulty breathing, heart palpitations, irregular and/or fast heartbeat, increased blood pressure, tremors or shaking movements, anxiety, nervousness, rapidly changing mood, problems with memory, blurred vision or other vision changes to name a few. Many drugs interact with Provigil which include over-the-counter medications, prescription medications, nutritional supplements, herbal products, alcohol containing beverages, and caffeine. The use of Provigil needs careful supervision. Provigil may affect concentration, function or may hide signs that an individual is tired. It is recommended that until an individual knows how Provigil affects him/her, they may not drive, use machinery, or do any activity that requires mental alertness.

Drivers being prescribed Provigil should not be qualified until they have been monitored closely for at least 6 weeks while taking Provigil. The treating physician and the medical examiner should agree that the Provigil is effective in preventing daytime somnolence and document that no untoward side effects are present. Commercial motor vehicle drivers taking Provigil should be re-certified annually.

What medications disqualify a CMV driver?

A driver cannot take a controlled substance or prescription medication without a prescription from a licensed practitioner.

If a driver uses a Schedule I drug identified in 21 CFR §1308.11 (§391.42(b)(12)) or any other substance such as amphetamines, a narcotic, or any other habit-forming drug, the driver is medically unqualified. Methadone use is disqualifying, as is any anti-seizure medication used for the prevention of seizures.

There is an exception: the prescribing doctor can write that the driver is safe to be a commercial driver while taking the medication. In this case, the Medical Examiner may, but does not have to certify the driver. The medical examiner has two ways to determine if any medication a driver uses will adversely affect safe operation of a CMV:

1. Review each medication — prescription, non-prescription, and supplement.

2. Request a letter from the prescribing doctor.

Can an employer have a policy requiring employees to disclose their drug use?

There are no FMCSA regulations prohibiting such a policy, and §382.213 of the CDL-driver drug testing rules authorizes employers to require the disclosure of therapeutic drug use. However, it is recommended that the employer consult with a legal professional for guidance on complying with medical privacy laws.

Can a CMV driver be disqualified for using a legally prescribed drug?

Although the driver may have a legal prescription, he/she may be disqualified if the medication could adversely affect the driver's ability to drive a CMV safely.

Can a driver be qualified if taking prescribed medical marijuana?

No. Drivers taking medical marijuana cannot be certified.

Cardiovascular

If a driver had a Myocardial Infarction (MI), followed by coronary artery bypass graft (CABG) several months ago, should he/she have an ETT (exercise tolerance test) as recommended in the MI guidelines but not in the CABG guidelines?

Medical examiners should follow the most current clinical guidelines; therefore, after an MI, drivers should obtain an ejection fraction and ETT before returning to work and, because of the CABG, should be kept off work for 3 months (not 2 as for MI) to allow time for sternal wound healing.

What is a satisfactory exercise tolerance test?

A satisfactory ETT requires exercising to a workload capacity of at least six METS (through Bruce Stage II or equivalent) attaining a heart rate of >85% of predicted maximum (unless on beta blockers), a rise in SBP >20 mm Hg without angina, and having no significant ST segment depression or elevation.

Stress radionuclide or exercise echocardiogram should be performed for symptomatic individuals, individuals with an abnormal resting electrocardiogram, or individuals who fail to meet the ETT requirements.

Can a driver who takes nitroglycerine for angina be certified?

Yes. Nitroglycerine use is not disqualifying. The examiner may require an evaluation by the treating cardiologist to make sure the angina is stable.

How soon may a driver be certified after coronary artery bypass grafting (CABG) surgery?

The driver should not return to driving sooner than 3 months after CABG, to allow the sternal incision to heal. The driver should have clearance from a physician (usually a cardiologist), a resting echocardiogram with an LVEF >40% after CABG, and be asymptomatic with no angina.

Can a driver be qualified if he/she is having recurring episodes of ventricular tachycardia?

Drivers with sustained ventricular tachycardia (lasting > 15 seconds) should be disqualified. Drivers experiencing non-sustained V-TACH should be evaluated by a cardiologist to determine the effect on the driver's ability to drive safely, treatment, and if the underlying cause of the ventricular tachycardia is disqualifying (see cardiovascular guidelines for complete review).

Can I drive a commercial vehicle after having angioplasty/stents inserted into my heart?

Yes. Drivers who have uncomplicated, elective Percutaneous Coronary Intervention (PCI), with or without stenting, to treat stable angina may return to work as soon as one week after the procedure. Criteria for return to work after PCI include:

- Examination and approval by the treating cardiologist;

- Asymptomatic;

- No injury to the vascular access site;

- ETT three to six months post PCI. In the CMV driver this requires exercising to workload capacity of at least six METS, attaining a heart rate >85% of predicted maximum (unless on beta blockers), a rise in SBP >20 mm Hg without angina, and having no significant ST segment depression or elevation. Stress radionuclide or echocardiography imaging should be performed for symptomatic individuals, individuals with an abnormal resting echocardiogram, or those drivers who fail to obtain the minimal standards required from the standard ETT;

- Annual medical qualification examination;

- Negative ETT at least every other year (criteria above) and tolerance of all cardiovascular medication.

IX. Reference

The driver should not experience orthostatic symptoms, including light-headedness; a resting SBP <95 mm Hg systoloc; or a systolic blood pressure decline >20 mm Hg upon standing.

Hypertension

Is the medical examiner required to repeat the entire physical exam if the driver is only returning for a blood-pressure check?

Yes, if the examiner completed an exam and issued a certificate to the driver. Once an exam is completed and a certification decision has been made, the examiner may not issue another certificate at a later date — or extend the original expiration date — without completing an entirely new exam.

If a driver with hypertension has lowered his/her blood pressure to normal range, lost weight, and is off medications, can he/she be certified for 2 years?

This is the medical examiner's decision.

Diabetes

May a driver who has non-insulin treated diabetes mellitus (treated with oral medication) be certified for 2 years?

In all cases, clinical judgment is required. The medical examiner decides if the driver's diabetes is adequately controlled, which determines certification, length of certification, or disqualification. FMCSA guidelines recommend performing annual examination for vision, neurological function, and cardiovascular disease, including hypertension. In general, the diabetic driver should have annual re-certification exams.

Kidneys and Dialysis

Can drivers on dialysis be certified?

According to the FMCSA, drivers who are on dialysis cannot drive. Certification, however, is left to the examiner to decide.

Is proteinuria disqualifying?

Depending on the amount, protein in the urine (Proteinuria) may indicate significant renal disease. The medical examiner may certify, time limit, or disqualify a commercial driver with Proteinuria. The decision is based on whether the examiner believes that Proteinuria may adversely affect safe driving regardless of the examiner's decision. The driver should be referred for follow-up.

May a medical examiner qualify a driver who has blood in his urine?

The medical examiner decides to certify, time-limit, or disqualify. The decision to certify a driver is determined by whether the examiner believes that the blood in the urine affects the ability of the commercial driver to safely. Regardless of whether the CMV driver is certified, the medical examiner should document referral to a specialist or the driver's primary care provider.

Respiratory

Can a driver on oxygen therapy be qualified to drive in interstate commerce?

In most cases, the use of oxygen therapy while driving is disqualifying. Concerns include oxygen equipment malfunction, risk of explosion, and the presence of significant underlying disease that is disqualifying, such as pulmonary hypertension. The driver must be able to pass a Pulmonary Function Test (PFT).

What are the criteria used to determine if a driver with lung disease can be certified?

At the initial and follow-up examination, the medical examiner can use general certification criteria:

- What are the effects of the lung disease on pulmonary function?

- Is the disease contagious?

- Can the driver safely use therapy while working?

- Can the driver safely perform both driving and ancillary duties?

- Is the disease progressive? A driver with a pulmonary disease that may progress or affect their ability to drive safely should be certified at least annually.

Certification for most chronic lung diseases is based on the clinical course. The examiner must decide if additional testing is required. The medical certification form states that the examiner may need to order a chest x-ray or pulmonary function tests.

Other Conditions

Is sleep apnea disqualifying?

Drivers should be disqualified until the diagnosis of sleep apnea has been ruled out or has been treated successfully (see the FMCSA bulletin regarding sleep apnea in the Reference area). As a condition of continuing qualification, it is recommended that a CMV driver agree to continue uninterrupted therapy such as CPAP monitoring and undergo objective testing as required.

A driver with a diagnosis of (probable) sleep apnea or a driver who has Excessive Daytime Somnolence (EDS) should be temporarily disqualified until the condition is either ruled out by objective testing or successfully treated.

Narcolepsy and sleep apnea account for about 70% of EDS. EDS lasting from a few days to a few weeks should not limit a driver's ability in the long run. However, persistent or chronic sleep disorders causing EDS can be a significant risk to the driver and the public. The examiner should consider general certification criteria at the initial and follow-up examinations:

• Severity and frequency of EDS,

• Presence or absence of warning of attacks,

• Possibility of sleep during driving,

• Degree of symptomatic relief with treatment, and

• Compliance with treatment.

Is Meniere's Disease disqualifying?

Meniere's Disease, a condition associated with severe and unpredictable bouts of dizziness (vertigo), is disqualifying. This recommendation can be found in the *Conference on Neurological Disorders and Commercial Drivers*.

Is narcolepsy disqualifying?

The guidelines recommend disqualifying a CMV driver with a diagnosis of narcolepsy, regardless of treatment because of the likelihood of excessive daytime somnolence.

Can a driver who has a condition that causes excessive daytime sleepiness be certified?

Narcolepsy and sleep apnea account for about 70% of EDS. EDS lasting from a few days to a few weeks should not limit a driver's ability in the long run. However, persistent or chronic sleep disorders causing EDS can be a significant risk to the driver and the public. While most of these diseases are usually disqualifying, The examiner should consider these general certification criteria at the initial and follow-up examinations:

• Underlying condition causing the EDS,

- Severity of and frequency of EDS,

- Presence or absence of warning of attacks,

- Possibility of sleep during driving,

- Degree of symptomatic relief with treatment, and

- Compliance with treatment.

After the initial evaluation, the examiner can decide if additional testing is required. Generally, drivers with excessive EDS need further evaluation to determine the cause and certification.

Waivers and Exemptions

What is a waiver? An exemption?

A waiver is temporary regulatory relief from one or more of the FMCSRs given to a person subject to the regulations, or a person who intends to engage in an activity that would be subject to the regulations. A waiver provides the person with relief from the regulation for up to 3 months.

Section 391.64 provided waivers to CMV drivers who were in the initial vision program in the early 1990's. By 11:59 P.M. March 21, 2023, drivers that used the federal vision exemption or waiver study program must be qualified under the alternate vision standard. On March 22, 2023, section 391.64 will no longer be in effect, and any medical examiner's certificate issued under a §391.64 or the federal vision exemption program are void.

An exemption is temporary regulatory relief from one or more of the FMCSRs given to a person or class of persons subject to the regulations, or who intend to engage in an activity that would make them subject to the regulation. An exemption provides the person or class of persons with relief from the regulations for up to 2 years, but may be renewed.

Who can issue a waiver or exemption?

Only the FMCSA grants waivers or exemptions for certain medical conditions if the individual is otherwise qualified to drive. The medical examiner cannot grant waivers or exemptions. Section 381.205 of the FMCSRs allow the driver to request a waiver if one or more of the FMCSRs prevent the driver from operating a CMV or make it unreasonably difficult to do so, during a unique, non-emergency event that will take no more than 3 months to complete.

How long will it take the agency to respond to my request for a waiver?

The agency will issue a final decision within 180 days of the date it receives your completed application. However, if you leave out required information, it takes longer to complete your application.

Can I get an exemption from any medical standard?

A CMV driver may apply for an exemption from any of the standards. Exemptions are granted only in those instances where the driver can show that safety would not be diminished by granting the exemption. See §381.300.

How do I request a waiver/exemption?

For exemptions from the federal vision, hearing, and epilepsy/seizure standards, refer to the FMCSA's website for application details. For exemptions or waivers from other standards, refer to §381.210 and §391.310

Who should I contact if I have questions about the status of my application for a vision exemption?

You should contact the Office of Bus and Truck Standards and Operations, Federal Motor Carrier Safety Administration, 1200 New Jersey Avenue SE, Washington, DC 20590. The telephone number is (703) 448-3094.

IX. Reference

Who should I contact if I have questions about the information I am required to submit to the FMCSA to obtain a waiver or exemption?

You should contact the Office of Bus and Truck Standards and Operations, Federal Motor Carrier Safety Administration, 1200 New Jersey Avenue SE, Washington, DC 20590. The telephone number is (703) 448-3094.

Online Resources

E-Mail Contacts

For information about federal medical exemptions:

- medicalexemptions@dot.gov
- fmcsamedical@dot.gov

For information about driver medical qualification:

- fmcsamedical@dot.gov

FMCSA Websites

Federal Motor Carrier Safety Administration (FMCSA):

- www.fmcsa.dot.gov

FMCSA Medical Programs:

- www.fmcsa.dot.gov/regulations/medical

National Registry of Certified Medical Examiners:

- http://nationalregistry.fmcsa.dot.gov

FMCSA Driver Exemption Programs and Applications:

- www.fmcsa.dot.gov/medical/driver-medical-requirements/driver-exemption-programs

FMCSA Medical Review Board:

- www.fmcsa.dot.gov/mrb

FMCSA Medical Expert Panel/Evidence reports:

- www.fmcsa.dot.gov/regulations/medical/reports-how-medical-conditions-impact-driving

Medical Conference Reports:

- www.fmcsa.dot.gov/regulations/medical/medical-reports-archive

Cardiovascular Resources

Cardiovascular Advisory Panel Guidelines for the Medical Examination of Commercial Motor Vehicle Drivers:

- www.fmcsa.dot.gov/sites/fmcsa.dot.gov/files/docs/cardio.pdf

Respiratory Resources

Tech Brief: A Study of Prevalence of Sleep Apnea Among Commercial Truck Drivers:

- Available from: https://rosap.ntl.bts.gov/

Other

Americans with Disabilities Act:

- www.ada.gov

Health Insurance Portability and Accountability Act of 1996 (HIPAA):

- www.hhs.gov/hipaa/

REFERENCE

FMCSA Contact Information

FMCSA Service Centers

The Federal Motor Carrier Safety Administration (FMCSA) maintains Service Centers, to which official correspondence may be directed, and Field Offices, where the safety investigators for each state are located. The field offices are also referred to as "divisions." Each state has one Field Office, which is where the Division Administrator for that Field Office is located. The staffs at these offices are ready and willing to answer questions and help anyone who is interested in improving commercial vehicle safety.

Eastern Service Center

Fallon Federal Building
31 Hopkins Plaza, Suite 800
Baltimore, MD 21201
(443) 703-2240
Fax: (443) 703-2253

Connecticut, Delaware, District of Columbia, Maine, Maryland, Massachusetts, New Hampshire, New Jersey, New York, Pennsylvania, Puerto Rico, Rhode Island, Vermont, Virginia, Virgin Islands, West Virginia

Southern Service Center

61 Forsyth St., SW, Ste. M40 (Midrise)
Atlanta, GA 30303
(404) 327-7400
Fax: (404) 327-7349

Alabama, Arkansas, Florida, Georgia, Kentucky, Louisiana, Mississippi, North Carolina, Oklahoma, South Carolina, Tennessee

Midwestern Service Center

4749 Lincoln Mall Dr., Ste. 300A
Matteson, IL 60443
(708) 283-3577
Fax: (708) 283-3579

Illinois, Indiana, Iowa, Kansas, Michigan, Minnesota, Missouri, Nebraska, Ohio, Wisconsin

Western Service Center

Golden Hills Office Centre
12600 W. Colfax Ave., Ste. B-300
Lakewood, CO 80215
(303) 407-2350
Fax: (303) 407-2339

Alaska, American Samoa, Arizona, California, Colorado, Guam, Hawaii, Idaho, Montana, Nevada, New Mexico, North Dakota, Northern Mariana Islands, Oregon, South Dakota, Texas, Utah, Washington, Wyoming

Note for Canadian and Mexican Carriers:

Canadian carriers should contact an FMCSA division (state) office in AK, ME, MI, MT, NY, ND, VT, or WA.

Mexican carriers should contact an FMCSA division (state) office in AZ, CA, NM, or TX.

REFERENCE

FMCSA field offices

Alabama
Federal Motor Carrier
Safety Administration
520 Cotton Gin Rd.
Montgomery, AL 36117-2018
(334) 290-4954
Fax: (334) 290-4944

Alaska
Federal Motor Carrier
Safety Administration
222 W 7th Ave., Ste. 518
Anchorage, AK 99513
(907) 271-4068
Fax: (907) 271-4069

Arizona
Federal Motor Carrier
Safety Administration
230 North 1st Ave., Ste. 200
Phoenix, AZ 85003-1725
(602) 379-6851
Fax: (602) 379-3627

Arkansas
Federal Motor Carrier
Safety Administration
Room 2527 Federal Bldg.
700 W. Capitol Ave.
Little Rock, AR 72201
(501) 324-5050
Fax: (501) 324-6562

California
Federal Motor Carrier
Safety Administration
1325 J St., Ste. 1540
Sacramento, CA 95814-2941
(916) 930-2760
Fax: (916) 930-2778

Colorado
Federal Motor Carrier
Safety Administration
12300 W. Dakota Ave., Ste. 130
Lakewood, CO 80228
(720) 963-3130
Fax: (720) 963-3131

Connecticut
Federal Motor Carrier
Safety Administration
450 Main Street, Suite 524
Hartford, CT 06103
(860) 659-6700
Fax: (860) 659-6725

Delaware
Federal Motor Carrier
Safety Administration
College Business Park
1203 College Park Dr., Ste. 102
Dover, DE 19904-8703
(302) 734-8173
Fax: (302) 346-5101

District of Columbia

Federal Motor Carrier
Safety Administration
1200 New Jersey Ave, SE
Maritime Administration
Mail Stop 5 / Rm. W26-
417
Washington, DC 20590-
0001
(202) 366-4000
Fax: (202) 219-3546

Florida

Federal Motor Carrier
Safety Administration
3500 Financial Plaza, Ste.
200
Tallahassee, FL 32312
(850) 942-9338
Fax: (850) 942-9680

Georgia

Federal Motor Carrier
Safety Administration
61 Forsyth St., SW
Ste. 3B15 (Bridge)
Atlanta, GA 30303
(678) 284-5130
Fax: (678) 284-5146

Hawaii

Federal Motor Carrier
Safety Administration
300 Ala Moana Blvd., Rm.
3-239
Box 50226
Honolulu, HI 96850
(808) 541-2790
Fax: (808) 541-2702

Idaho

Federal Motor Carrier
Safety Administration
1387 Vinnell Way, Ste. 341
Boise, ID 83709
(208) 334-1842
Fax: (208) 334-1046

Illinois

Federal Motor Carrier
Safety Administration
3250 Executive Park Dr.
Springfield, IL 62703-4514
(217) 492-4608
Fax: (217) 492-4986

Indiana

Federal Motor Carrier
Safety Administration
575 N. Pennsylvania St.,
Rm. 261
Indianapolis, IN 46204-
1520
(317) 226-7474
Fax: (317) 226-5657

Iowa

Federal Motor Carrier
Safety Administration
105 6th St.
Ames, IA 50010-6337
(515) 233-7400
Fax: (515) 233-7494

REFERENCE

Kansas

Federal Motor Carrier
Safety Administration
1303 SW First American
Pl., Ste. 200
Topeka, KS 66604-4040
(785) 271-1260
Fax: (877) 547-0378

Kentucky

Federal Motor Carrier
Safety Administration
330 W. Broadway, Rm. 124
Frankfort, KY 40601
(502) 223-6779
Fax: (502) 223-6767

Louisiana

Federal Motor Carrier
Safety Administration
5304 Flanders Dr., Ste. A
Baton Rouge, LA 70808
(225) 757-7640
Fax: (225) 757-7636

Maine

Federal Motor Carrier
Safety Administration
Edmund S. Muskie
Federal Bldg.
40 Western Ave., Rm. 411
Augusta, ME 04330
(207) 622-8358
Fax: (207) 622-8477

Maryland

Federal Motor Carrier
Safety Administration
George H. Fallon Federal
Building
31 Hopkins Plaza, Ste.
750
Baltimore, MD 21201
(443) 703-2360
Fax: (443) 703-2374

Massachusetts

Federal Motor Carrier
Safety Administration
50 Mall Rd., Ste. 212
Burlington, MA 01803
(781) 425-3210
Fax: (781) 425-3225

Michigan

Federal Motor Carrier
Safety Administration
315 W. Allegan St., Rm.
219
Lansing, MI 48933-1514
(517) 853-5990
Fax: (517) 377-1868

Minnesota

Federal Motor Carrier
Safety Administration
Warren E. Burger Federal
Building & US
Courthouse
316 North Robert St., Ste.
244
Saint Paul, MN 55101
(651) 291-6150
Fax: (651) 291-6001

Mississippi

Federal Motor Carrier
Safety Administration
100 West Capitol St., Ste.
1049
Jackson, MS 39269
(601) 965-4219
Fax: (601) 965-4674

Missouri

Federal Motor Carrier
Safety Administration
3219 Emerald Ln., Ste.
500
Jefferson City, MO 65109
(573) 636-3246
Fax: (573) 636-8901

Montana

Federal Motor Carrier
Safety Administration
2880 Skyway Dr.
Helena, MT 59602
(406) 449-5304
Fax: (406) 449-5318

Nebraska

Federal Motor Carrier
Safety Administration
100 Centennial Mall
North, Rm. 406
Lincoln, NE 68508-5146
(402) 437-5986
Fax: (402) 437-5837

Nevada

Federal Motor Carrier
Safety Administration
705 N. Plaza St., Ste. 204
Carson City, NV 89701
(775) 687-5335
Fax: (775) 687-8353

New Hampshire

Federal Motor Carrier
Safety Administration
James C. Cleveland
Federal Office Building
53 Pleasant St., Ste. 3300
Concord, NH 03301
(603) 228-3112
Fax: (603) 223-0390

New Jersey

Federal Motor Carrier
Safety Administration
5 Independence Way, Ste.
250
Princeton, NJ 08540
(609) 275-2604
Fax: (609) 275-5108

New Mexico

Federal Motor Carrier
Safety Administration
2440 Louisiana Blvd., NE
Ste. 520
Albuquerque, NM 87110
(505) 346-7858
Fax: (505) 346-7859

REFERENCE

New York

Federal Motor Carrier
Safety Administration
Leo W. O'Brien Federal
Bldg., Rm. 815
Clinton Ave. and N. Pearl
St.
Albany, NY 12207
(518) 431-4145
Fax: (518) 431-4140

North Carolina

Federal Motor Carrier
Safety Administration
310 New Bern Ave., Ste.
468
Raleigh, NC 27601
(919) 856-4378
Fax: (919) 856-4369

North Dakota

Federal Motor Carrier
Safety Administration
4503 N. Coleman St., Ste.
204
Bismarck, ND 58503
(701) 250-4346
Fax: (701) 250-4389

Ohio

Federal Motor Carrier
Safety Administration
200 N. High St., Rm. 609
Columbus, OH 43215-2482
(614) 280-5657
Fax: (614) 280-6875

Oklahoma

Federal Motor Carrier
Safety Administration
300 N. Meridian, Ste. 106
North
Oklahoma City, OK
73107-6560
(405) 605-6047
Fax: (405) 605-6176

Oregon

Federal Motor Carrier
Safety Administration
The Equitable Center
530 Center St., NE, Ste.
440
Salem, OR 97301-3740
(503) 399-5775
Fax: (503) 316-2580

Pennsylvania

Federal Motor Carrier
Safety Administration
215 Limekiln Rd., Ste. 200
New Cumberland, PA
17070
(717) 614-4060
Fax: (717) 614-4066

Puerto Rico

Federal Motor Carrier
Safety Administration
Torre Chardón
350 Chardón St., Ste. 207
Hato Rey, PR 00918
(787) 766-5985
Fax: (787) 766-5015

Rhode Island

Federal Motor Carrier
Safety Administration
20 Risho Ave., Ste. E
East Providence, RI 02914
(401) 431-6010
Fax: (401) 431-6019

South Carolina

Federal Motor Carrier
Safety Administration
1835 Assembly St., Ste.
1253
Columbia, SC 29201-2430
(803) 765-5414
Fax: (803) 765-5413

South Dakota

Federal Motor Carrier
Safety Administration
1410 E. Highway 14, Ste.
B
Pierre, SD 57501
(605) 224-8202
Fax: (605) 224-1766

Tennessee

Federal Motor Carrier
Safety Administration
640 Grassmere Park, Ste.
111
Nashville, TN 37211
(615) 781-5781
Fax: (615) 781-5780

Texas

Federal Motor Carrier
Safety Administration
903 San Jacinto Blvd.,
Ste. 1100
Austin, TX 78701
(512) 916-5440
Fax: (512) 916-5482

Utah

Federal Motor Carrier
Safety Administration
2520 W. 4700 S., Ste. 9B
Salt Lake City, UT 84129-
1874
(801) 288-0360
Fax: (801) 288-8867

Vermont

Federal Motor Carrier
Safety Administration
87 State St., Rm. 305
P.O. Box 338
Montpelier, VT 05601
(802) 828-4480
Fax: (802) 828-4581

Virginia

Federal Motor Carrier
Safety Administration
400 N. 8th St., Ste. 780
Richmond, VA 23219-4827
(804) 771-8585
Fax: (804) 771-8670

REFERENCE

Washington

Federal Motor Carrier
Safety Administration
724 Columbia St., NW,
Ste. 200
Olympia, WA 98501
(360) 753-9875
Fax: (360) 753-9024

West Virginia

Federal Motor Carrier
Safety Administration
700 Washington St. East
Geary Plaza, Ste. 205
Charleston, WV 25301
(304) 347-5935
Fax: (304) 347-5617

Wisconsin

Federal Motor Carrier
Safety Administration
1 Point Place, Ste. 101
Madison, WI 53719-2809
(608) 662-2010
Fax: (608) 829-7540

Wyoming

Federal Motor Carrier
Safety Administration
2617 East Lincolnway,
Ste. F
Cheyenne, WY 82001
(307) 772-2305
Fax: (307) 772-2905

Note for Canadian and Mexican Carriers: Canadian carriers should contact an FMCSA Field Office in AK, ME, MI, MT, NY, ND, VT, or WA. Mexican carriers should contact an FMCSA Field Office in AZ, CA, NM, or TX.

SUBJECT INDEX

This subject index is designed to help you quickly locate information in the **DOT Medical Exams: The Complete Guide.**

SUBJECT	PAGE

A

F

R

S